Purple Stew

or

My Kid's Got What?!

Purple Stew

or

My Kid's Got What?!

compiled by

Karen Tompkins

Cranberry Tree Press
Windsor, Ontario, Canada

Cranberry Tree Press
Windsor, Ontario, Canada

Canadian Cataloguing in Publication Data

Tompkins, Karen, 1966–
Purple stew, or, My kid's got what?

ISBN 1-894668-05-7

1. Joubert syndrome—Popular works. 2. Joubert syndrome—Patients—Biography. I. Title. II. Title: My kid's got what?.

RJ486.T48 2001 616.8 C2001-900012-X

This book is dedicated to the three women who inspired the Joubert Syndrome Foundation: Cheryl Duquette, Mary Van Damme, and Joanne Eastman, as well as all the Board members and volunteers who make a difference in our childrens' lives everyday.

Special thanks to Dorothy Mahoney whose work and life have always been an inspiration for me.

And of course, Kevin, without whom none of this would have ever been possible. Thanks for sharing the journey.

Ingredients

Making a purple stew. Whip whip whip whip.
Making a purple stew. Scoobi-doobi-doo.
With purple potatoes and purple tomatoes
And YOU! How do you do?
Fancy meeting you in a purple stew.

—*Children's game*

I usually order clear soups: chicken noodle, minestrone. I want my meals to be like my life: safe, well known, comforting because they're common. But still, I always entertain the notion of something more exotic when I go to order. Perhaps seafood chowder, Cajun gumbo—but Purple Stew??! The idea intrigues me but my appetite for comfort always brings me back to chicken noodle, predictable and easily identifiable chicken noodle.

So, I place my order. Occasionally I wonder briefly why some people would ever order stew. The ingredients always appear to be vague representations of their former selves. I'm never sure what I'm going to experience until it's been tasted. What would I do if I bit into a big chunk and then discovered I didn't like it?

I have to admit, the few times I've been served stew at a friend's house it has been a pleasurable experience. Aunt Evelyn's stew was one of these. A perfect blend of vegetables and herbs that made me relax and enjoy the surprising harmony of flavours. But it wasn't enough to prompt me to order it voluntarily, and I definitely wasn't ready for the purple kind. Perhaps no one is.

Letter From Your Child

Dear Mom and Dad,

I may not be able to put in words how I feel about you, but I want to let you know how much I appreciate all you do for me.

In the months before I was born, you had dreams of a perfect, precious baby. After my birth, doctors told you about all the things that were wrong with me and about all the problems I would have. Thank you for still thinking of me as your perfect, precious baby. I know I am cherished.

My first doctors gave you a grim view of my future. They told you all the things I would never do and all the things I could never learn. Thank you for not taking them seriously! Because you held fast to hope and decided to tackle the impossible, I have been able to accomplish things no one ever expected.

Thank you for all the sacrifices you have made on my behalf. Because of all the expenses, you have gone without different things—renovations on an outdated kitchen, the trip to Paris, a new winter coat. You decided that the old car will make do for a couple more years. And yet you don't complain. You tell me I'm your priceless treasure and that you're the richest people in the world.

Thank you for all the time and hard work you devote to caring for me and teaching me. It takes months and sometimes years for me to learn things that other kids do naturally. But you keep persevering, even when you're tired, even when I'm uncooperative, even when there are no signs of progress. No one will ever know how hard it is for you, but I know, and God sees the way you give of yourselves so unselfishly.

You are my heroes. You're stronger and more courageous than Hercules and Zena, the Warrior Princess. You not only have wisdom, but insight to find in me all the special qualities no one else sees. You represent me in a society that might otherwise turn away. You are my voice, a persistent advocate in my behalf. You have taken on the world for me.

Please do something else for me. Take care of yourselves and take time to relax. Contrary to previous predictions, I could be around for a long time, and I will continue to need you. Taking care of yourselves is one of the best things you can do for me.

And so, Mom and Dad, for all the things that remain unspoken, but not unnoticed...thank you. The next time you see my radiant smile, just know it's a reflection of the love you bestow so freely. I am richly blessed through you. I love you.

...Now sign this letter with love from your son or daughter. The next time you feel discouraged, please remember that you have enriched the life of your child more than you will ever know. And whether you realize it or not, you have even made an impact on our world. May God bless you all richly as you continue to raise your precious children.

Joanne Eastwood
4th International Joubert Syndrome Conference
June 24-28, 1998

Part One

Erin's Story

It's been six years almost to the day and I feel as if I'm right back where I started. Sitting beside my daughter who is hooked up to more wires and machines than I can count while people in pastel cottons scurry busily around, brings back more emotions in me than I want to remember. I'd worked hard to forget the terror, the confusion and the anguish of those first days when I realized I might never know the baby we wanted so desperately. After two miscarriages, to have come so far only to lose another child; I was just as afraid of losing myself to the overwhelming feelings of despair as I was of losing her.

Erin entered this world and she was perfect. She still is perfectly Erin, but at the moment of birth she also fit my ideal. When they laid her on my stomach, she sang a cute little "ah" with her first exhale. She scored a nine, a nine, and then a ten on her APGAR ratings (a test that rates the health of newborns) and as a mark oriented teacher, I was proud and relieved. By the next morning, my image of perfection was not being realized. Because of a staff shortage, there was no one to help me learn how to nurse my new daughter and I refused to give her a bottle. Kevin remarked that her breathing was irregular but the doctor's called it "periodic breathing—quite common in preemies" (Erin was born at thirty-eight weeks and weighed eight and a half pounds—not quite preemie standards!)

I never really registered Kevin's concern at that point. Perhaps it was the thirteen hours of difficult labour. But I think I was still so enthralled that she was here! My little Erin with perfect fingers and toes, chubby little cheeks and a button nose. She was everything I had dreamed of. I held her and changed her; rocked her and sang to her. Early in the pregnancy I had purchased a tape of Disney lullabies and learned three of them ("Baby Mine" is still a family favorite) and I was overjoyed to be finally using them. I was thrilled with all the little details of my new mom routine: memorizing her face and hands, inhaling her new-baby scent, choosing an outfit for her first picture. I was oblivious to anything that didn't fit into the perfect little world in my head.

I never noticed a thing...except I couldn't get a handle on the nursing. Erin wouldn't latch on and when she did, she couldn't sustain it. But the hospital was busy and noisy and I figured it was my fault. By Friday, she still couldn't nurse and was developing jaundice. I consented to water to keep her from dehydrating under "the lights".

Then came the early morning Saturday feeding. The nurse and I worked for an hour and a half at getting Erin to latch on to feed, but to no avail. Erin was extremely lethargic and neither of us clued in that there was more to it than that. It was the last time I saw the Erin of my dreams. Later that morning the nurses found her blue in the nursery, physically stimulated her to get her breathing again and placed her in NICU where a battery of tests would begin. I then took a good look at my real daughter Erin. And I discovered that she was ill and no one could tell me why.

Everyone always assumes that their child will be like everyone else's. According to women I've talked to, everyone also thinks at some point "what if". But there is no way to prepare for the reality of a child with special needs. It truly is an overwhelming experience. All along, you have fantasized and pictured yourself with your newborn; troubleshooting many roadblocks before the baby was even born to be better able to cope when the need arises. Then the entire situation changes. Not only are all your fantasies null and void, the pictures which take their place are often depressing. I started to remember when I was in grade school and called the kids who went to a nearby vocational school "nummy-nums". Why? That's what everyone else called them. When I was growing up, the boy next door had Down's Syndrome. He was older than me by about ten years and much bigger, or so it seemed to my six year old eyes! We often played together: baseball with a large green plastic bat, bike riding up and down the sidewalk on our half of the block or sitting on the porch and talking. But I was always afraid of him. Sometimes he would hurt me—not purposefully, but as a toddler does out of excitement for the game. I insisted that he sit on the bottom step of the porch while I sat at the top out of harm's way and close to the door so I could run in if necessary.

Yet I still chose to play with Donald. I never told him to go away when he came over. I remember scolding other kids on the block for being cruel to him. But I NEVER went to his house and invited him out to play.

When I was in my late teens, my boyfriend had a little brother with Cerebral Palsy and vision problems. His speech was severely compromised and at eight years old he was struggling to walk with braces and crutches. He preferred to scootch around on his bum. What I remember most about Ian is his smile. It covered his entire face and I couldn't help but respond to it. His mother told me that I should work "with kids like Ian" and I was immediately flattered and repulsed by the suggestion. I told her I liked dropping by and playing with Ian on my terms when I felt like it but I couldn't see myself doing "that sort of thing" from nine to three everyday, ten months a year. I was sure I didn't have that in me. I also thought about my reactions as an adult to "challenged" people— mental or physical. Curiosity, pity, even disgust. Would I feel that for my own baby? Would others?

Then came the grieving. Erin would not be the ideal I had pictured. The rational part of me recognized that no child would have been. Your children are their own people. Even in the womb they move when they want to, not when it is convenient for you. At some point, in months or years, Erin would have expressed her own opinions and needs and I would have deferred to her personality and allowed her to develop it. But this was different. It's not so much that I wasn't ready for her to be her own person so much as I was afraid she wouldn't fit my loose definition of a person: someone who learns as they grow in order to one day be self-sufficient and possibly help someone else on the same journey. Would she ever be independent? Could I be there forever if she needed me to?

And so I grieved for the child that wasn't. And I grieved for me: the parent yet to be. I had never raised a child. What if she were more than I could cope with? I don't believe the statement "God gives special kids to special people." I didn't do anything to deserve Erin (no matter if I thought she was a gift or punishment). And surely my tiny precious Erin didn't deserve all these tests and tubes. And so who could guarantee that I'd be enough for her. I know that I'm not alone. There is Kevin, but he feels the same things differently. Could we do this?

Erin was also very ill. Her reflexes (grasping, sucking, etc.) were vanishing. At times, she looked comatose. They ran test after test. Nothing. And everyday I let the doctor call the shots, asked few questions and never consciously prayed.

How oblivious I was! Every four hours, day and night, I would put on my slippers and go down to NICU, take Erin out of the isolette and try to get her to nurse, sometimes for an hour! Then I would give her back to the nurse who would feed her and put her back under the "the lights" (I had consented to formula, bottles, anything they wanted by this time.) All the time I was there I would sing to Erin, chat and joke with the nurses, anything to keep from feeling the panic rise in my throat.

She might die. It was a litany that played in the back of every moment of my being. *She might die.* And I smiled and joked and created a routine of mindless details.

Six days after Erin was born, a nurse suggested I go for a walk with Kevin. I hadn't realized I hadn't seen the sun for a week. Time had become meaningless. Hours had just been a period of waiting to see Erin again.

I tried to stay away from NICU. I wasn't able to hold her because of the jaundice (the less time she spent in the lights, the longer it would take to "get better"). And I was afraid of all the tubes and wires and beeps. Afraid of really understanding what they were for and afraid of giving way to the panic that was always there, ready to scream out of my throat if I let my guard down, even for a moment.

So I tried to remain detached from the reality of it all. I would recite all the names of the tests of the day and the results the morning report brought in. But it was like lines in a play, and not a well performed one. The words were hollow and the smile was forced. But my love and connection to Erin was growing and swelling despite her absence from my arms and eyes, even as the panic increased and threatened to take all the available space inside me.

Then the doctor ran out of ideas and I took charge of my daughter's future. It was at that moment, seven days after her birth that I accepted her totally, but not yet unconditionally. The doctor wanted to transfer her to another local NICU. Kevin and I asked what they would do there that he couldn't do here. He wisely stated "if I knew, I'd be doing it." We insisted that if she be moved, they send her to London where there were teaching hospitals and one of the best facilities in the province, some two hundred kilometers away. He tried to dissuade us but we were firm in our decision and he made the arrangements.

I'm still not sure how I got through those first few weeks. I know my faith in my religion deepened to a new, stronger level. Perhaps I already had that strength, and just didn't realize it until then.

I remember talking to the nurses at the Windsor hospital the day Erin was transferred to London. I had had a few courses in Developmental Psychology in university and it suddenly clicked that there was a good possibility that Erin's problem was developmental. I talked to the nurses about my theory, that since she was losing her innate reflexes, something was desperately wrong in her brain. I wondered about this out loud and that perhaps my body had worked for her in the first days after birth and now that she was supposed to take over, her brain wasn't able to do the job. The three women in the room exchanged glances and told me "You are an intelligent woman. You should always trust your instincts." Then one of them hugged me fiercely and told me "Now, go fight for your daughter and make them transfer her to London."

When Kevin finally arrived (that one morning he was fifteen minutes later than usual, an eternity had passed and hundreds of lives had changed), I quickly ushered him into a room and caught him up on news. Then I started talking about all the things that had happened in the last nine months and that maybe I had wished this on her. He held me and assured me it was untrue and although rationally I believed him, I still wasn't sure.

* * *

Kevin and I had started trying for a family in September of 1991. By Mother's Day I was worried that maybe we couldn't. I was at my in-laws for Mother's Day Brunch and as the only childless female, I offered to cook the pancakes. As I was doing this, Kevin's mother came in the kitchen and cheerfully said in a hopeful voice "Maybe next year, you won't have to do any cooking!" at which point I started sobbing. When Kevin noticed, he was very concerned; after all, I don't cry often and my body was shaking with choked off sobs. I had just finished my cycle and felt like I would never get pregnant. I began to regret those times before I was ready to start a family that I was afraid of being pregnant. Now, I was a wreck because I wasn't!

The next Friday, I was driving home from work and looking forward to having my niece and her friend over for a visit. Suddenly, a pain shot through my abdomen and lower back. It took my breath away and I had to concentrate to keep control of the car. I figured I was having bowel problems. Sure enough, I got home and went to the toilet. But I also discovered a few spots of blood. I thought it was strange, being only two weeks since my last period but the flow had been shorter than usual so maybe my body was just "finishing up". So, I cleaned up and sat on the couch with Kevin. I had a few more cramps but they weren't as severe. A few minutes later I want back to the washroom and the flow was very heavy. I immediately knew something was wrong but was too afraid to tell Kevin. I sat with him for a few more minutes then blurted out the whole story. I've always felt better after sharing my fears with Kevin. He has an incredible calming effect on me. So he bundled me off to emergency where they ran blood work and did an exam and we were told I was pregnant, for the time being. The doctor said I was having a miscarriage and that I was to stay overnight and they would run more tests in the morning to see if my body would save the baby or if it was already too late. They talked to us about the percentage of pregnancies that end in miscarriages (ten percent) and the number of women who have them (one in four). And although we were sad, a part of us rejoiced because indeed we could get pregnant!

Six weeks later I was pregnant again and we told everyone!! Then at eight weeks I started having some spotting, spent a few days in bed and went back to work. There was no pain, no red blood, just a few brown spots occasionally. The doctor said there was nothing to be concerned about but after three more weeks, I demanded an ultrasound.

The day of the test came and Kevin and I were so enthralled to see the outline of our baby on the screen that the technician had to repeat three times that the baby wasn't moving. Well, the babies in the ultrasound pictures in the book never moved either!! I didn't know this one was supposed to.

We were devastated. Suddenly, this little person that I was protecting all these weeks was a dead thing inside my uterus and I couldn't wait for them to get "it" out of me. I had to wait three days for a D&C. I chose to go to work until then. I figured I couldn't just sit around with my thoughts, I'd just wallow in ice cream and get even more depressed.

I felt the loss of that baby deeply. I had a friend who was due the same time as me and it became awkward to be around her. We both had so many things we wanted to say but couldn't. And as it is with good friends, we didn't have to. But I grieved for that baby even after Erin was born. I thought of him (I think it was a boy...I've thought all my pregnancies were boys until they were in my arms and proved otherwise!) on what would have been his day of birth and calculated how old he would have been until about his fourteenth month. By then I had two live little girls to contend with which didn't leave much time for wistful wonderings. Now I only think of him occasionally.

Two months later I was pregnant again. (I had never fallen off of my bicycle much as a child so didn't really see the drawbacks of getting right back on!) This time, we told no one. At five weeks, I experienced some pains in the left side of my abdomen. Off we went for another ultrasound. Kevin and I barely talked about it. I think I may have told him how I felt: that if we lost this baby I would need to take a break from trying. Physically and emotionally, three in six months would be more than I could take.

There wasn't an outline of any baby on the screen. I

panicked. Kevin gripped my hand tighter. There was only this flicker-blip. Then the technician commented that the baby's heartbeat was strong and regular and pointed to the flicker and we both resumed breathing and cried.

We followed the pregnancy closely and other than constant indigestion and pain in my hips after the sixth month, the baby was doing fine. (I found out later the hip pain was sciatic problems. Oh, to have been at a chiropractor then! But I just thought it was a "normal" pregnancy thing!)

I was so happy to be having a baby it made up for how much I hated being pregnant. When people asked me if we hoped for a boy or a girl, I would answer, "It doesn't matter." And they would go on the next line of the age-old script, "That's true. As long as the baby is healthy." But I always changed the script there and added the line, "No. As long as it's a baby!"

And on that day in July, when my fantasy world collapsed, those words rang in my head. Had I known? Was it a premonition? Or did I wish it.

It was probably none of these. I've always been a practical person and don't "put much stock" in fate. My mother helped me to see the clearest path in any situation and it's served me well. (A sad coincidence: my mother experienced many consecutive miscarriages in the era before ultrasounds and hormone therapy. And I was ready to give up after two. How strong she was. I've respected that about her more since Erin than in all the years before.) I enjoy bringing order to chaos—that's probably why I teach high school. That, and I've always taken on more jobs/projects than a sane person should. I like to be busy, I like to be organized and I like to be in control. And even though I was trying to be in control of Erin's care, I was floundering in a sea of panic and unknown fear. I couldn't even organize what to be afraid of first because we still had no idea what was wrong.

* * *

So we followed Erin to London. They took her by air-ambulance and we drove. It was the longest drive of our lives. We stopped to put the house in order on the way as we had no idea when we would be back. I remember going into Erin's room all clean and perfect with the Teddy Bear Picnic wallpaper and colourful striped curtains. I vowed I wouldn't return without her and by doing so, admitted that I might not.

We emptied the mailbox that was filled with best-wishes and congratulations: cards from friends and family. We cried a great deal and prayed that we would be able to introduce these people to Erin soon. The two hour drive seemed an eternity and while we were driving, the doctors in London had already begun their battery of tests. And the list was impressive.

No one could have prepared me for the reality of the St. Joseph's NICU. We walked inside to a lengthy sign-in and wash-up procedure and a barrage of forms. But the real jolt was the walk from the first double doors to Erin's bed. There were three basketball-court size rooms with several private areas built in, and every six feet, another crib or isolette with several machines and monitors, all beeping, buzzing and blipping. A row of desks piled high with thick binders took up the centre corridor. And there was a sea of pastel uniforms.

And of course, there were babies. Some were so small, my wedding ring would have fallen off their thighs.

Another was distended and waxy-yellow—I thought it was a training doll until I realized the monitors were registering a real heartbeat. I tried not to look at the other babies. Aside from it being overwhelming, I thought it would be rude. There wasn't much room for privacy and I didn't want to intrude on the only place anyone had to be a family with their child.

We were there for ten days. At the time it felt like years; now, it was a matter of minutes. Every day was the same: new tests and results (always "within normal range"); trying to nurse Erin; trying to keep from thinking, crying, screaming... always singing and rocking and cuddling; never knowing if this "goodnight" would be the last and not believing that it could. We looked forward to going home so things could get back to normal, but we never knew what normal was. During that time in the NICU, Erin had more tests than I could count. Her grand total by age seventeen days was two spinal taps; one MRI; one CAT scan; two EEGs; Xrays of heart and lung; upper GI barium swallow; blood work for metabolic disorders, several dozen viral infections, blood gases and many other reasons I never registered; IVs for medications administered "just in case"; and many people looking at her, holding her, talking about her, hypothesizing- and no one knowing.

In the early hours of July 30th (why does everything happen pre-dawn?) the nurses observed three moderate seizures. She was given a "loading dose" of Phenobarbital then switched to Dilantin, another anti-seizure medication. That day she had her second spinal tap, an EEG and several rounds of blood work. Around midday, we were asked to join the team in The Quiet Room. Kevin's parents were there for a visit and we left them with Erin and went out of the NICU into a small room done in dove gray, country blue and rose. There were three love seats, two wing chairs and a box of Kleenex on every end table. I knew they were going to give us difficult news.

They said that some of the tests they were running were for various infections which attacked the brain, the most common of these being herpes. We were told that since Erin had appeared fine at birth and had degenerated to the point where seizures had begun, it was very likely that it was a viral infection. If it was herpes, they had a medication to control it and they wanted permission to start the drug right away as the test results would take several days and they didn't want to wait that long. They asked me if I had had herpes. I told them no, that I rarely ever have cold sores on my mouth! But I didn't dismiss the possibility. I asked if it was possible to have herpes and never have any symptoms and they said yes. When we asked about treatments for other viral infections that target the brain, they said there were none. Erin would have to fight those on her own. They then politely asked if we had any other questions and we calmly asked about making arrangements for a crib side baptism for the next day and they left the room. Kevin and I looked at each other and lost it.

We had been so good keeping ourselves in check but this was exactly what we had been dreading for the last ten days. I apologized over and over for doing this to our baby. Kevin had not been my first sexual partner and I immediately regretted that fact. I sobbed and screamed and apologized. And then we prayed that it really was herpes since that was the only one they could control. Then we laughed at the irony of that prayer. Kevin handed me more Kleenex, told me he loved me, that he did not blame me, that it wasn't my fault and gave me a big hug. We cried some more then cleaned up and went to tell his parents. (They were beside themselves by this time. They had seen the medical team return and we were not with them.) I spent the rest of the day making arrangements for Erin's baptism. I called everyone I knew to be a prayerful person and encouraged them to call all their friends. That weekend we had hundreds of people from seven denominations praying for Erin and our family.

The next week was like a drug-induced dream. Erin's tests came back slowly through the week...and all were within normal range. The EEG showed some slight epileptic spikes in the temporal lobe but epilepsy was not a diagnosis. She did not have herpes. She did not have a viral infection targeting her brain. She continued to take Dilantin. Erin started to be aware of her environment more often, cried during her bath, started being removed from monitors...even started nursing (a bit). By August 7, one week later, we were allowed to bring her home. And still, no one could tell us why anything in these past two and a half weeks had occurred.

With Erin at home, I began to try to find a normal rhythm in our lives. In the morning, I would put Erin in her snuggly pack and walk for a bit. (This was getting increasingly difficult as she got heavier. By September, she was ten pounds and my hips were giving out when I lifted her. I got myself to a chiropractor and within weeks felt enormous relief.) When we got back from our walk, I would place her (still sound asleep) in her swing-o-matic and jump in the shower. I had the shower, hair-to-toes, done in two minutes flat. The whole time I was in there, I would have these imaginary headlines running through my head: "Baby Dies 'Cause Mother Takes Shower." "Selfish Shower Leads to Baby's Demise." I would scrub and rinse even faster, then run out to see if she was still pink. (The swing itself wouldn't fit in our small bathroom and she would wake up if I put her in a stationary seat.) Oh the joys of a first baby!

On August 20, Erin's "periodic breathing" took a new turn. Her respiratory rate became extremely accelerated and she began eating voraciously. We went to the pediatricians who sent her for chest x-rays and blood gases. Both were normal. Then we went to London to see Dr. Apple, the pediatric neurologist from her hospital stay. Erin's breathing was "normal for her" by the time we completed the two hour drive and all testing and observations done there were reported to be "within normal range". So we went home and thought "that was a weird experience" and went back to adjusting to our new lives.

Of course, our lives were nowhere near what I had anticipated as normal. Erin went to Windsor one or two times a week (two-hour round trip) for blood work and pediatric appointments. We had EEGs in London every sixth week for three visits; she needed to have an audiology exam to ensure there were no side effects from several of the medications she had been on in hospital, a VON came to our house once a month to check on her progress; and any time anything out of the ordinary happened, I was on the phone with questions.

Yet, I don't think I was overprotective. True, I rarely put her down, but she slept in her own crib in her own room without an apnea monitor, just a regular nursery monitor to pick up her breathing (she was a very noisy breather for many years). By September, I was convincing Kevin we should have another child right away. Although no one had officially said anything, I still felt that Erin might have developmental problems. We knew that she had neurological problems which had caused the seizures and seemed to be affecting her breathing so it wasn't much of a leap to assume her general development might be delayed. My argument was that Erin needed an older sibling to be our eyes and ears at school, to help her learn and do things that we might not be able to teach her. And, I couldn't see how I would cope with a three year old who possibly couldn't walk and be nine months pregnant. Looking back, I know we entertained the notion that Erin's problem might be genetic, but we didn't dwell on it. By now, I was a firm believer in the power of positive thinking and pure, blind faith. But I did worry at times.

November 1, 1993 was a difficult day. Just as I was beginning to feel comfortable in my routine and began forming a sigh of relief.....BANG! Reality took another bite. When the VON arrived that day, she administered a developmental assessment (The Denver Scale) and told me that Erin was behind in several areas. We were due to see the neurologist in two days so I agreed to discuss her results with him. It wasn't that this report was unexpected, I just didn't want to accept it.

That evening, Erin had an apneatic episode. It was about six o'clock in the evening. Erin was lying in our big, blue Lazy Boy chair, sound asleep and Kevin and I were talking (probably about the Denver Scale results). I glanced over at her and her lips were blue. I cried out, picked her up quickly, held her at arm's length and gave her a quick shake. She took a big breath but did not wake up. So, we called her name and poked her a couple of times until she woke up fully and smiled. By this time, she was pink and happy, but we went to the Emergency Room. After relating Erin's story for yet another ER doctor, all blood work and tests came back normal so we went home and lay in bed listening to her breathing.

Our visit with Dr. Apple confirmed our suspicions since day ten: Erin's development was delayed. He told us her last EEG showed her electrical impulses were lower than normal with one side being lower than the other and that led him to believe there may also be a cognitive delay.

As I read these words in my notes (I kept a medical log for the first year to help remember what everyone was telling me. It made doctor and ER visits much less stressful) I don't remember registering the idea of a cognition problem. I knew she wasn't doing things she was supposed to at this age but I never believed she wasn't thinking things. I always assumed that she thought just like I did; her body just didn't always get the right message. I never realized how accurate my assumptions proved to be.

So Erin began seeing an occupational therapist, a physiotherapist, had consults with a speech therapist, received regular visits from an Infant and Family Worker (Leslie Wagner was my angel for the next two and a half years. She was supportive, helpful, creative—and an excellent listener. She was always able to keep me focused and make me feel competent and special. Thanks, Leslie!) and began receiving monetary assistance for all the long distance phone bills, driving and parking and eventually, an in-home worker. For that next year, we drove to Windsor two or three times a week, London one or two times every three months, had in-home appointments two to four times a month plus the occasional ER visit. It was a good thing that I was already applying for my next maternity leave when I returned to work from Erin's! I would have had to take a leave just to chauffeur her to all her appointments!

Sarah Dorothy Tompkins was born August 9, 1994; eight and a half pounds; pink and perky. She nursed immediately, was strong and alert and did everything according to the textbook, except sleep. She was much too busy for that. So between Sarah's body clock and Erin's breathing episodes... well, I'm still catching up on sleep. There were many times in that year that I reflected on how lucky I was that I had always been a person with a large amount of energy. I wasn't always sure where it was coming from or if it would run out but I thanked God I had it.

Sarah was the perfect companion for Erin. Erin watched Sarah's natural development and tried to keep up with her. She became more active and had more incentive to reach for the toy, to roll over or scoot to get the toy back after Sarah took it away.

But those first few months were very difficult. Sitting in our big blue chair nursing Sarah, I would watch as Erin tried over and over to reach her toy that had fallen out of her hands. I would try to ask her to wait until Sarah was done eating, but Erin was only thirteen-months old, an age where waiting is not a highly developed skill. So I would move down on the floor and nurse Sarah while playing with Erin. This wouldn't have been too bad, but with all the interruptions (including constant kisses and hugs from her doting sister). Sarah rarely had a good, filling meal, and consequently wanted to eat every one or two hours around the clock! By Thanksgiving, we were bottle feeding.

Walks were a big thing that first year with two children. We had a beautiful tandem stroller (a gift from my parents) and lived in a picturesque small town with one stoplight and two parks. We would pack up the stroller with Erin in the front and walk for thirty to sixty minutes, singing and talking all the way, unless Erin was having a "bad day", which was happening more and more frequently.

One concern was her eating. When we introduced solid foods at six months, Erin seemed to really enjoy it. She didn't have a great deal of control over her tongue, jaw or lips so eating was very messy but not traumatic. We began doing oral massage, using a Nuk brush, and experimenting with different spoons.

I was reminded of the first time her speech therapists came for a home visit when Erin was five months old. I was giving her a bottle and talking with Arlene and Kris. We chatted for about thirty minutes and Erin fell asleep after eating approximately two ounces of formula. Kris asked if this was a typical feeding for Erin and I said yes: after all, I thought infants were supposed to only sleep, eat and get rid of it, right? Wrong. Apparently, most infants drink several ounces in less than twenty minutes and still have energy left to play. But not my Erin. We started searching for "the perfect nipple" for Erin: soft enough that she could suck easily but hard enough that she could feel it was there. It also had to reach just past the middle of her tongue but not too long as to trigger the gag reflex. She also had a very high palate and the nipple should stimulate that as well. We tried several types and brands (none of which were returnable/refundable) and finally ended up with one she liked and met most of the criteria. We used these until she was three years old when she was adept enough at drinking from a sippy-cup that I felt she would get enough liquids in her day without too many clothing changes!

At some point during the solid food experiments, Erin began clamping down on her tongue until it was blue/black and all the food would come oozing out the sides of her mouth encased in saliva. We would scoop up all the food as it oozed out, press down on her tongue until her jaw released and deposit the whole mess back in her mouth. All the while we would be giving her verbal cues of our expectations (Open wide! Num,num,num! Swallow! Open wide! etc.). After about an hour, she would have eaten a small jar of baby food and the person feeding her was ready for a nap. We didn't go out to eat much during that phase!

Over the year we tried different textures, temperatures, etc. I became concerned about her nutritional intake, which seemed to consist of cookies, crackers and whatever baby food she actually swallowed. Toddler foods in all popular brands were out of the question. The mix of chunks and sauce were difficult for her to separate: if she swallowed the sauce, she choked on the chunks and if she gummed on the chunks, the sauce poured out of her mouth. Campbell's Vegetable Soup was a mainstay. Undiluted with mashed up crackers, it was a homogenized blend of mush that she managed well. I began making muffins (Robin Hood mixes) with jars of baby food vegetables (just add water and bake a little longer than the directions call for) and these seemed to work well, too. Cheesies and Froot Loops were offered often, more from a therapeutic aspect than nutrition. As we got to more solid foods, things improved but I'm not sure when the tongue biting actually stopped. I just know that we go to restaurants now without any problems.

Erin's breathing was still a major concern. The accelerated breathing at one and three months had graduated to twenty-four to thirty-six hours of erratic breathing during which the breath rate was accelerated (hyperpnea) followed by a cessation of breath (apnea) from which she would heave a deep noisy breath and resume the accelerated rate. And all of this was arrhythmic. There was no beat to her breathing. Some breaths were short, others long; some pauses were more pronounced than others. A deep inhale was not always followed by a full exhale.

Her behaviour was affected during these "episodes" as well. She was unable to complete tasks she had already mastered (e.g.. holding and manipulating toys) and her moods were much more demanding. These episodes occurred every three to four days.

We talked to the pediatrician and to the neurologist, Dr. Apple, and were told that "special kids react to things in special ways". They then suggested that since her episodes seemed to escalate at night, perhaps she was simply reacting to a wet diaper or needed a hug. Kevin and I knew that Erin had a wet diaper every night, not just every third or fourth. We also hoped that she wanted hugs as frequently as a new diaper. We had already tracked every environmental cause possible (foods, detergents, perfumes on other people she had occasional contact with and when we saw them, weather systems, bowel function, etc.) and found no clues there. So we sought a second opinion from a developmental pediatrician, Dr. Brown.

We were well prepared for this visit. I had hand delivered all previous documentation regarding Erin's health and therapies and included a video tape of her at various stages of an "episode". I also included this report:

Erin normally:

has a pleasant disposition
good attention spans
scheduled routine which her body initiates
sleeps soundly (10–12 hrs per night, 1–3 hour nap)
plays well "by herself" for extended periods (up to one hour)
is not very vocal
demanding and fussy when hungry or tired

During an "episode":

breathing becomes accelerated and erratic
has little attention span (3–5 minutes)
becomes very vocal—predominantly "ah" and squealing
rarely sits alone (will throw herself back toward the floor)
wants to nibble at a bottle frequently but won't stay with it for more than 5 minutes
very demanding and fussy for most of the day
sounds like she is having a nightmare while in sleep—very restless
will quiet down briefly when held then becomes "fussy" again
needs a constant change of "low input" stimulation
very disorganized (more pronounced than normal)
not a lot of fun to be with!

How an "episode" usually progresses:

EVERY 3–4 days (very little variation), Erin will not

nap well. She will become excited for no apparent reason (accelerated breathing, squealing, active movements). She still eats normally and goes to bed at her normal time.

Then, around 10 pm–12 am, she becomes very restless in sleep (sounds like she's having a nightmare). There seems to be a cycle involved—> breathing accelerates; restless movement; squealing—> all three build until either we pick her up or sometimes she just stops. She then starts again from the "beginning" 5–20 minutes later. When we pick her up, she doesn't really wake up (unless she is having a very bad time of it and then she wakes and cries).

She starts her morning earlier than usual and crying. She won't nap long through the day and when she does sleep, the same pattern occurs as observed in the evening. Even when awake, a cycle of accelerated breathing, restlessness and squealing occurs, but not as pronounced as in sleep.

She goes to bed later than usual at night, but she calms down through the night and is back to her normal self by morning (she tends to sleep more the next day!)

Other comments and observations:

Her breathing is not as affected now as it was in Jan./Feb. She still pauses/stops breathing and then "catches up" during an episode but not as severely as before. She sighs a great deal in normal sleep.

We can't find any trigger for these "episodes". We've looked at internal causes (teething, gas, etc.) and external (weather systems, foods, changes in routine). NOTHING we've looked at occurs every 3–4 days!

When the day came for Erin's appointment (three weeks after Sarah was born), we were told that in his opinion, Erin would walk by the time she was two and a half, that verbal communication was not far away and that even if we could make a diagnosis, there would be no "magic pill" for her to take to make her just like everyone else. When we pressed him to explain the episodes that we described, he was unable to help us. He said, "Even if we could think of other tests to run, we wouldn't know how to treat her." He then submitted the following conclusions in his written report:

1. I do not know the diagnosis. With the early history of respiratory irregularities one might think of the Joubert Syndrome but she is neither severely retarded nor microcephalic nor does she have a brain stem or cerebellar anomalies usually found in this mysterious condition.

2. Furthermore, I am not convinced that the items within the history which seem important to the parents are necessarily of great significance. The evidence that the reported sleep disturbances are invariably or necessarily followed by a breakdown in behavioral integrity the next day is scant. Sometimes the behaviour precedes rather than follows the disturbed sleep. Furthermore, the video tape of her sleep did not reveal anything which was definitely abnormal. The patterns of increased movement, change in respiration and quasi purposive rolling are very reminiscent of what we see in REM sleep. Certainly these episodes did not appear to be seizures.

3. The parents have generally felt that only with a specific diagnosis would they be able to answer the child's needs. In discussion today they said "maybe this is just the way she is". They accept that she has had some brain injury, and I reviewed the features which might make us think that this was closer to the brain stem, although apparently there are some cerebral insults on the neuroimaging which I have not seen.

4. The parents are clearly shopping around and may never be satisfied until they are given some very specific label or explanation. In counseling today I suggested that even if there were a specific label it was quite unlikely that this would help in rehabilitation or provide some miraculous surgical or medical intervention.

I was furious. This wouldn't be the only time that I'd be angry with a member of the medical profession, but it was the first, and I'm still trying to get rid of the bitter taste of condescension. How dare he dismiss me as an overprotective parent with unrealistic expectations! I *was* "shopping around" but I did not consider that a negative trait. I was pursuing every avenue I had to find a way to relieve my daughter's suffering. I believed that these patterns of erratic breathing were interfering with Erin's development. One day every three to four days she lost skills. The next day she would be exhausted from the previous twenty-four to thirty-six hours. That left only one or two days for normal, effective learning to take place before the cycle began again. Of course I wanted a "specific label or explanation". I'm her mother. That is my job. So we began the process for a third opinion.

In Ontario, Canada in the 1990's, it took several months to get in to see a specialist and so we waited three months to see another pediatric neurologist, Dr. Calla. In the meantime, Kevin and I had many discussions about how many "second opinions" we would pursue. Were we going to travel the province until we got an answer? Would we go to the USA? Who would we trust as a final expert opinion? We had discovered that Dr. Brown worked closely with Dr. Apple and had in fact discussed Erin's case with him prior to his examination. Dr.

Apple had just happened to be at Brown's office while he was watching the video we sent. Kevin and I both felt that this had biased his thinking. Dr. Brown did not examine Erin with an open mind. He had a working theory based on Dr. Apple's opinion that he was going to prove or disprove. When a colleague tells me something about a student that will be joining my class, I find it impossible to generate my own first impression. We felt this to be true in our case as well, but it was hard to know if we were thinking objectively or indeed simply "shopping" for a feel-good label to tell our friends.

November came and the appointment with Dr. Calla proved anticlimactic. After more talk and blood work, forms and questions, we were told that she had no idea what Erin's diagnosis could be. She was very polite and sympathetic and she gave some ideas to explore, but her answer was the same as the others. But it was OK. I felt we had done the right thing in seeking this opinion and although it didn't change Erin's situation, it at least eased my mind a bit.

That fall/winter was bittersweet for Kevin and me. We settled into a comfortable (if sleepless) routine filled with babies and bottles, cuddles and giggles. Kevin was between jobs and I was still on maternity leave so we were able to go on many walks as a family: to the park, window-shopping, around the neighbourhood. Even going to get the mail was an adventure!

Christmas that year was memorable. Friends and family received many handmade treasures and baked goods (when did I sleep?) and we had plans for many guests over the holidays. On Christmas Eve, Kevin came down with a nasty flu bug and a very high fever. We canceled our Christmas day plans and snuggled in for the night.

We woke the next morning and helped the girls rip all that beautiful paper and played with the boxes. Kevin crawled back upstairs to bed and within the hour, both girls had temperatures and were vomiting! Merry Cleanup! I managed to avoid the bug but spent most of New Year's in bed catching up on sleep!

Sleep was something I decided I needed to do more often as I prepared to return to work. Being a mom was the other thing.

From the time Erin was seven days old, I had been her "primary care nurse", the person responsible for all her medical decisions, all information gathered and given, scheduling, recording, paying workers: the list went on. I couldn't read a book to her without ticking a mental checklist of daily activities and new accomplishments. Even my memories of those first years are filled with names and lists and symptomology. I needed to let go of the details and feel again. I wanted to learn to be a mom.

The transition was very difficult. I am an educator with a minor in developmental psychology. I had once entertained the idea of becoming a physiotherapist for special needs kids. And although it was not the path I chose, it was easy to act as if I was Erin's therapist. Being able to use "therapy speak" which turned Erin into a client, allowed me to be detached, to look at things objectively. I rationalized that it helped me make the right decisions but really it just allowed me to not feel.

It's not that I didn't love Erin! I love her very much. But I didn't want to examine the emotions I had surrounding being her mom and everything that meant and would mean. But that wasn't a new problem for me.

One of the main reasons I had always been so busy even before I had Erin was to not have time to think too much. There were many "unresolved issues" from my teenage years which although I understood, I hadn't taken the time to deal with effectively. And even though I had changed a great deal in those first few weeks of Erin's life (a deeper faith in God; a slowing down of self; more patience; and a better understanding and appreciation of differences) I had fallen back into the habit of "busy-ness" to mask my avoidance.

The therapists involved with Erin would shake their heads in disbelief when I tried to prepare them for the changeover of power. Although I would be the one to bring Erin to her therapy sessions, the in-home worker would be carrying out the prescribed activities. They would smile and say, "But you'll still be doing them, too! You won't stay out of it. You're an involved mom. You'll always be a part of the equation." I know what they meant and in a sense all they said was true but I needed to redefine my role in my mind. Yes, I would always be informed of what was happening with her therapies and I would ensure that she received everything she needed. But I wanted to read to her because I'm a mom who likes to read, not because it's 3:30 on Tuesday and she should practice turning pages and identifying colours!

Dr. Apple called late one Sunday night to review Dr. Calla's report. She had suggested looking into Erin's elevated lactate levels and was wondering if we wanted him to do the follow-up or were we planning on going to Dr. Calla. Since Dr. Apple had initiated the idea of pursuing Dr. Calla's report and he knew Erin's complete history, Kevin and I decided we would like to continue working with him. And I'm glad we did. Since that time, our visits to Dr. Apple have become yearly reviews of Erin's progress, a continued dialogue of hypothesis and information which I look forward too. And afterward, Erin and I go out for a special lunch and shopping. (Of course, I'm hoping that as she gets older, a place with a waiter will be more enjoyable than McDonald's!)

Dr. Calla had made several suggestions, some of which we had already followed up on. She had ordered "chromosomal prophase banding studies" and I admired her willingness to explore other areas. While Drs. Apple and Brown had dismissed metabolic disorders as a probability, Dr. Calla agreed that it was possible and made arrangements for lab work to be done during Erin's next episode. When Dr. Apple contacted us that night, it was to tell us that all the tests had come back normal except one—Erin's lactate levels were high. He said there were several reasons for having high levels of this nature, one of which was inadequate sampling and he would therefore like us to come up to London for a more controlled sample to be taken. Of course, we agreed.

The lactate level in your blood is the byproduct of activity. If you have run a long race or a very fast sprint, your lactate levels would rise slightly for a short time. Erin's were usually elevated and sometimes three times the "normal" level. They often had trouble taking blood from her—poking and prodding with the tubing tight on her arm and Erin screaming the whole time—and that alone could be the reason for the elevated lactate. Or, she could have a mitochondrial disorder.

I spent a few days on my March break that year taking a course on Internet surfing. (It amazes me how steep my learning curve in computers was that summer! When I started the course, I didn't even know how to "log on". I suppose necessity is the mother of many things.) I learned that the mitochondria is the part of the cell that makes energy out of nutrients for the cell to do its work. There were many enzymes involved in this process and some could be synthetically produced and injected to compensate. In other words, IF Erin did have a mitochondrial disorder, AND we could pinpoint which enzymes were missing in the chain we MIGHT be able to help her with a specific enzyme therapy.

We also decided that Erin should have another MRI just to be sure that nothing had changed and then schedule a muscle and nerve biopsy to check for mitochondrial problems after that.

During this time, we were also battling "baby-sitter-from-hell syndrome" as I had gone back to work full time in February, 1995. First, there was Lucy who lied about little things. When I reminded her that the girls were to only have a treat after lunch and preferably apples or cheese and crackers, she pronounced that she NEVER gave the girls anything like chips or pop. (well, unless she was putting her own big butt on the booster chair, how were chip crumbs getting between the booster and the kitchen chair it was strapped to?). And the time I found one of the kids' books shoved at the back of the shelf with its pages ripped (obviously the work of an excited Sarah) and asked if Sarah had gotten hold of another book. She professed, "No. Sarah never rips books!" Well, I love Sarah, but she is a very normal child and even at that young age already had a very deep love for books, just not the kind of love we wanted her to have! So, since I had caught her in two lies in one week, I wasn't sure what I could trust her to do or say anymore and we let her go.

Then we got Mary. Mary was actually a housekeeper who was tired of cleaning other people's houses for a living and having raised her own kids, figured she would switch to that. My house sparkled! But when I went to the local grocer's, the check out girl said, "I hear Erin's therapy went well this morning!" I tried not to let that bother me though, after all, we were living in a very small town at the time and that is part of the "charm" of small town life. A few weeks later though, a friend in town called and told me that she had witnessed Mary in the passenger seat of a car with my seven month old Sarah perched on her lap! (Erin had been at home with the in-home worker that morning.) Well, I must say I was an angry mama-bear! I called Mary and explained what I had heard and she confirmed it saying her husband was a safe driver. I said that I was sure he was but could they guarantee the safety records of all the other drivers on the road? That is why they are called accidents, after all. No one intends to smash a car in order to catapult a seven month old child through the windshield to land in front of an oncoming transport truck! I told her that I could no longer trust her judgment and to not return to work.

We were blessed to have Sharie (ironically, the friend who called me about Mary) come with her newborn and six year old and take care of the girls for the last three months of the school year. I enrolled them in the day care near my high school for the following September.

The night before the MRI was particularly stormy and snowy so I convinced Kevin to drive to London that night rather than be snowed in two hours away from the hospital in the morning. We had waited over six months for this test and I did not want to lose my spot. (Since Erin was not in a high-risk situation, the wait period was much longer—and we didn't demand it be scheduled earlier.) As it happened, Kevin reported the roads were bare a half an hour away from our house and the next day dawned clear and crisp!

Again, it was a Sunday evening when Dr. Apple called us with the results of the MRI. Erin was missing a piece of her brain! Since the MRI done at ten days of age had been reported as normal, I asked the obvious: "So. Are you telling me this is degenerative? Is something eating her brain? 'Cause she doesn't seem to be losing skills!" And indeed, this was not the case. Dr. Apple admitted that the first MRI "may have been misread" but that it was quite clear in these latest films. He then told me that he was now able to give a tentative diagnosis of Joubert Syndrome but since he had not been able to compare the two MRIs, he would not commit to a definite diagnosis. We then discussed the probability of continuing with the muscle and nerve biopsy. Joubert Syndrome also accounted for the hypotonia and muscle weakness [see Appendix A] but not for the lactate levels ... although the high levels could still be due to the difficulty in acquiring a sampling. Since he seemed hot to find a connection between Joubert Syndrome and mitochondrial disorders and Kevin and I wanted as much information as possible (and the mitochondrial thing actually had a "sorta cure") we agreed to proceed with the biopsy.

Now we had a name. And to be honest, it felt pretty anticlimactic, or maybe I was just stunned that the journey seemed...over. One of many ironies in my life is that in Dr. Brown's report "oh, so long ago" he mentions Joubert Syndrome but dismisses it since "she is neither severely retarded nor microcephalic". Today, we know that these symptoms are rarely present in people with Joubert's or not at all.

I received information about a parent's support group in the USA with a contact name in Michigan. Other than that, I didn't have much more new information: no therapy, no cure, no answers. Just a name for the syndrome and a name to call.

In retrospect, calling the Joubert Syndrome Parents-In-Touch Network (as it was called then) was the beginning of a two year transition for me from finding a name to "doing something about it." It was early evening in mid-June and Kevin was either sleeping or working and the girls were tucked into bed when I picked up the phone and called the contact name for the parents group: Mary Van Damme. She answered the phone and I introduced myself. I expected her to take my name and address and mail me out some flyers or something. Instead, we talked for almost an hour, comparing notes on development and diagnosis, sharing our fears for the future, answering my questions and offering a wealth of information. She told me of a conference taking place in Chicago in two weeks time, but with final exams going on, lack of money and being totally overwhelmed by all this new information, I didn't feel we could attend. But definitely when the next one came around in two years time, we would be there. Erin would be five then and we would have more definite questions. We also wanted to send copies of Erin's MRI films to Dr. Maria at the University of Florida. He had been doing research on Joubert Syndrome, and we wanted a final opinion on the diagnosis.

Mary did take my address but she didn't send a flyer; she sent pages of updated research (although much more has been done since then) and best of all, old newsletters that the Network put out quarterly. For the first time,

Kevin and I looked at pictures of kids and read stories by other parents and said, "That's just like Erin!" And it was wonderful to be able to really truly feel that she indeed was perfectly Erin and that we weren't alone anymore.

And we learned that the erratic breathing patterns were a major part of the Joubert Syndrome profile. I couldn't help but feel angry. If the first MRI had been read correctly, we would not have worried quite so much those past three years—and definitely would have spared her countless trips for blood work and surgery. (She did not have a mitochondrial disorder. It was the poor quality of the samplings that gave the inconsistent results.) But, I don't dwell on those things. I can't change it. It didn't make anything worse. Let's move on.

Prior to the last decade, very little was known about the brain. Most studies needed to be done in post-mortem situations which, by its nature, were usually a "worst case" scenario. Such was the case with Joubert Syndrome. First identified in 1969 by Dr. Marie Joubert in Montreal, Canada, the description was grim. These first articles talked about a high-infant mortality rate, usually before age five, severe mental retardation and minimal skill development. A very bleak outlook! I believe that there were many other cases of Joubert Syndrome then but the less severe cases were not recognized for two reasons. Primarily, in "those days", if your child was slow to develop but not medically fragile (no life threatening complications) you just accommodated for their needs, found him or her a job on the farm or around the neighbourhood and life went on. There wasn't the same demand for labels and slots as we seem to need now. Secondly, and perhaps more importantly, it was impossible to get an accurate picture of the brain! It wasn't until the advent of Magnetic Resonance Imaging (MRI) that we could detail with any accuracy what the brain might be missing while its owner was still living. As more live patients were diagnosed with Joubert Syndrome and earlier diagnosis began, the description of the syndrome changed. [see Appendix A]

The last half of 1996 was about as normal as our family had ever been. We went camping in July in Northern Ontario where it poured down rain for four of the six days we were there: two toddlers in a leaky dining tent being held and rocked by parents singing "Rain Rain Go Away" for hours on end. Picture perfect! Then, we drove to Ottawa and Montreal for overnight stays with family. In November we bought our first house and our December schedule was tight with packing, presents and parties.

The year 1997 dawned with bouts of the flu and plans for the future. We needed to make some decisions about Erin's schooling: public or Catholic; mainstream or sheltered; assistant or solo. We didn't want to underestimate her abilities but we didn't want her to flounder either. We finally decided on the local public school which housed the county's Community Living Program. She would attend a regular Junior Kindergarten classroom with no assistant but the school would provide a worker for toiletting and lunch time as Erin still wore diapers and had problems with zippers and containers. We also had feeding concerns as she would overstuff her mouth and choke on the contents. She would attend two full days per week and all her services (OT, PT, Speech) would continue at the Day Care for the year. It was also agreed that we would meet at Christmas and in April to reassess this situation. As it turned out, it was the best decision at the time but it did make it more difficult to have services in place for the next school year. At the IPRC (Independent Placement and Review Committee) meeting that spring, we were commenting on the wonderful progress she had made that year. I then rattled their brains a bit when I said, "Now it's up to you. She will be here full time with you providing all services. If she doesn't continue to make progress, it will be your fault." The looks of shock were priceless but I still feel it was a truthful statement. She grew by leaps and bounds at day care and made lots of wonderful gains. If that slowed or stopped, one of the major factors would be the school and their service provider!

That fall there were many cutbacks from the province in Special Education funding and it took four months to secure an assistant for fifty percent of Erin's school day. There were several times that I was ready to quit my job and home school her but as I wrote in my journal: (no, I do not keep one regularly, but I did that year!)

The easiest thing would be to quit my job and home school. But I don't believe that it's the best choice. By the time I brought her to all her doctor and therapy appointments, there would be no time for teaching! And she is very social—I want to keep her that way. Even though I anticipate tears (hers and mine) because of what other kids may say and/or do, the long term socialization would suffer if I home schooled. Her community would not have participated in her education and her peers would not know her on the street.

Just as Sarah was recovering from her Easter '97 Chicken Pox (she broke out two weeks to the day after

Erin's first spot!), Dr. Bernard Maria called from the University of Florida in Gainsville, Florida to confirm that Erin did indeed have Joubert Syndrome. We had purchased copies of both of the MRI films and mailed them down earlier in the year. We did a lengthy phone interview in which they asked if we could bring Erin in to their clinic. Well, it was cold and snowy that day and someone was asking me to go to Florida?!? Unfort unately between work and the expense, the answer had to be no. Dr. Maria said that it was quite clear to him on both films that Erin had the typical "molar tooth sign" found in Joubert Syndrome. That, along with the reported hypotonia and breathing difficulties, was enough to confirm a diagnosis.

So that was it. Erin's "thing" had a name. Everything was in a nice little box. Progress was being made in noticeable ways. We could now sit back and relax and be a normal family. But as the saying goes, "It's always something."

Our "something" was ears. Erin had many ear infections as an infant. Although not uncommon in children, I think it also had a lot to do with her low tone and her problems coordinating her suck/swallow mechanisms. The fluid in her ears never really drained and she was constantly on antibiotics to try and clear the infection. After the second course of antibiotics, she would invariably develop thrush and need a week on Nystatin to rebalance her body. She had been seeing an Ear, Nose and Throat (ENT) specialist since she was eighteen months for the problem. I didn't personally like Dr. Doan. The first time he met Erin he asked, "So why is she retarded?" I tried to be open-minded. After all, it was just a word and he was of a different generation and a different culture. But it was a word that grated on my sensibilities. Being a professional educator, I phrased my response carefully and replied that Erin's "growth was *delayed*, it had been *retarded*, because of an undiagnosed neurological problem." I then went on to talk about her history of breathing problems and brought the discussion back to her ears. I debated finding a new ENT but decided that his choice of words didn't necessarily reflect his medical knowledge.

Dr. Doan recommended tubes be inserted into her ears to assist with the drainage. The operation was very successful with no problems with anesthetic, which had been a concern with her low tone and erratic breathing.

The day of the operation was extremely stressful for my family. Ten days previous, my mother had gone in to the hospital to have a tumour removed from her colon. They suspected it was cancerous but felt that the surgery could successfully stop the cancer from spreading. They did biopsies of the liver and lymph nodes while they removed the tumour, which had grown in size since the last ultrasound had been done, just a few weeks earlier. My mother never recovered from the surgery. Twenty-four hours after surgery, she began having difficulties breathing due to an infection. She was placed on a respirator and given drugs to be put in a coma-like state in order for her body to heal faster and to prevent her body from fighting the respirator. But she was having problems as she could not regain consciousness when the drug was taken away. At the same time the results of the biopsies came back: cancer in all areas tested. So five days later, the doctor presented us with our options. Treat this present infection aggressively and when she regains her strength, begin aggressive treatment for the cancer.

These treatments could give her an extra year or two of life. And they could not assess what brain damage may have occurred due to the low oxygen during the onset of the infection. We decided to take the second option which was to take her off the drugs and the respirator and allow God and nature to take over.

Lois Mary Nagy died in the mid-afternoon of June 24, 1995. Erin's ear tube surgery was June 30th. I'm sure the hospital was astonished at this overprotective family pacing the halls during a fairly routine procedure. Aside from Kevin and myself, my dad and sister also came down to wait with us. Needless to say, we all were extremely relieved that there were no complications.

By August of 1997, the tubes were starting to work their way out. Three years is a long time on the same set of tubes and we felt lucky that they had worked so well. Kevin brought Erin to see Dr. Doan and he had Kevin hold Erin's head as he removed the tubes in his office. That night, there were a few spots of blood draining from Erin's right ear. A couple of days later, she had an infected discharge which required antibiotic drops to clear up. A hearing test done at the time and repeated in October had the same results: fifteen percent hearing loss in the right ear that had not been noted in earlier tests. We began looking for another ENT.

At our last appointment with Dr. Doan, I asked several times if the blood and ensuing infection were fairly common and each time, Dr. Doan evaded or ignored the question. I also had concerns about the size of Erin's tonsils. They were large, about the size of grapes, and often looked like they were blocking the majority of the throat. Dr. Doan had previously said he would like to wait until Erin "could chew gum" or at least until her third birthday before he did any surgery. Her speech pathologist also had concerns that the tonsils were interfering with formation of guttural sounds such as "k" and "g". When I brought this up with Dr. Doan again on what was to be our last visit, he began administering what I could only describe as a "homemade IQ test" consisting of pointing repeatedly to body parts and asking in a high pitch voice "What's this? What's this?" I told Erin that the doctor would like her to tell him what he was pointing to and with big eyes, she whispered, "Foot." He then stuck two fingers up in front of her face and screeched "How many? How many?" I asked Erin to tell Dr. Doan how many fingers he was holding up. She shrank back in her chair and shook her head no. He then sat back and smugly stated, "It is obvious the problem has nothing to do with the size of the tonsils." I gathered Erin and left his office.

In October, we went to see the new ENT. He told me that Erin was missing part of the ear drum in her right ear and if it did not close on its own, and it probably would not, they would do surgery to correct the problem when she was around ten years of age. His main concern was the size of her tonsils, especially with her low tone and history of apnea. He scheduled a sleep study with a tonsil and adenoid removal to follow.

The results of the sleep study were stunning. For an average of 44.5 minutes per hour, my baby was not breathing and many times her oxygen saturation count went down below 82%—the point at which soft tissue damage could occur. The tonsils and adenoids were removed promptly and the follow-up sleep study revealed a marked improvement: 12.8 minutes per hour with most due to central apnea and only a few due to obstructions to the airway. The best news was that there were only two times that the oxygen saturation levels were low. We then consulted a lawyer.

My desire to find a name had become my nemesis. Lawsuits are based on money; in this case, loss of potential income. If indeed Dr. Doan was negligent in not ordering a sleep study or not performing an adenotonsilectomy early enough, thereby allowing soft tissue damage, specifically brain damage, to occur due to long term apnea, then Erin was not reaching "normal wage earning capacity" because of that negligence. But we knew she had Joubert Syndrome and many people with Joubert's have global delays, including cognitive. And very few people with Joubert's live independently and are financially self-sufficient. There was no way to prove that Dr. Doan's inaction had caused Erin's ceiling of potential to be lowered. So out of pure survival instinct, Kevin and I have decided that no brain damage occurred and she would be no different had I left Dr. Doan's office that first day when he used antiquated, offensive terms.

All of this was taking its toll on our marriage. Although Sarah was "normal", she was a very assertive child and craved intellectual stimulation. She was constantly asking questions, wanting to be read to or play a game. She preferred to talk to you than play alone. She was exactly like me. In fact, there were many times when I looked at her and knew exactly what she was thinking and remembered feeling that way at that age. Erin was more like Kevin and they were completely foreign to me.

As in many couples, the things that had drawn us to each other were now things that irritated us the most. My energy at the beginning of our marriage now took me out of the home to work, to church or to community theatre. His "groundedness" kept him home watching TV and reading books. I talked out my thoughts until I came to a solution. He kept everything inside until he solved it in his head. We focused our energy on the kids, the house and the church and avoided talking about even the little things for fear of discovering how much we had grown apart.

By now, I was on antidepressants. I started on them shortly after mom died and had seen a counselor for a few months as well. I had been sexually abused by a family member outside of our home from the age of twelve to age sixteen and it had greatly interfered with my relationship with my mother when I was a teen. I remember my friends telling me that they really liked her and that she wasn't that bad. I felt so betrayed by them and retorted that they didn't have to live with her. But the truth was that she was a wonderful person. Yes, she had her faults but my anger was misplaced. I wanted her to know what that man was doing to me but I couldn't tell her because I didn't really understand it myself. So I was angry at her for not being able to read my mind and for not stopping the abuse that neither of us knew was happening.

I found out a great deal about myself during that counseling. Things about why I always needed to feel in control—because I could not control the abuse when I was young. And about why I was always afraid Kevin would suddenly change and become a different person—because my abuser professed care and then hurt me. And even why I would sometimes be mean and ignore the people I loved the most—because I did not love myself and wanted to prove that I was unlovable by turning everyone away from me.

Kevin and I had begun our marriage in a specific pattern and now I had changed and our children had changed us. There had been many other discussions about who did more work in the house and how to redivide those things ($80 a month for someone to come and clean twice a month did wonders for our marriage!). but on the long weekend in May, five years after that first miscarriage, Kevin and I finally talked about the state of our relationship. After many tears and hugs, I wrote this entry:

Kevin and I talked this weekend. It's very scary to know that he feels empty in our relationship too. We both still feel that there is "a light at the end" and we'll retire together... comfortable, happy and still intimate... but we need to find a way to work toward that.

So we spent the summer at a marriage counselor and we promised to spend more time together and save some energy for us.

But the cycle of silence and tears continued for two more years. Finally last year, we had a very open discussion about our individual battles with stress and depression and our future as a couple. By now, Kevin was working permanent midnights and between my work schedule and his sleep schedule, we would go days without spending more than thirty minutes together, often only five to ten minutes at a time.

It was during that discussion that we said it didn't matter how we got to this point, there was no blame of one being domineering or the other avoiding decisions. All that mattered was that we were both in a destructive pattern: neither of us could display that type of behaviour if the other didn't allow it. We agreed that we didn't dislike each other and that we were terrific parents. In fact, neither of us wanted to raise the girls alone and neither of us wanted someone else to help in that responsibility. So we agreed to focus on the kids and not "work" on our marriage anymore. There just wasn't anything left after the parenting was done for the day and my schoolwork returned to the briefcase to start another job. By deciding this, we discovered what many people already know: sometimes marriage is just about two people making a good home for their children. Since it no longer mattered that we made time to talk to each other, we started talking more about the little things, which has made it easier to discuss our feelings about the big things when they come up. Since it didn't matter if we had a perfect marriage, the marriage we did have became perfectly enjoyable. But it was a risk. Our apathy and despair could have forced us farther apart. But we both still hold that vision of us in our eighties taking walks together and holding hands over ice cream.

The next Joubert Syndrome Foundation (its new title now that they had attained nonprofit status) conference was quickly approaching. Held every two years, the 1998 conference was slated for Salt Lake City, Utah. Kevin and I were flying out with Erin, and Sarah was spending the week with Kevin's family. They've always been wonderful about taking one or both of the girls when we needed someone, and we definitely couldn't have made this trip without them.

It's wonderful how one child can bring an entire family or community together. Because of Erin's needs, many bonds were formed during her infancy, when just two parents weren't enough. For instance, Kevin's mom and dad, a constant source of support, still give regular updates to their friends who prayed for Erin the weekend of her baptism. As well, we made new friends who became family in Leamington and Wheatley. We never could have gotten through those first years without the Cats family—even now they are a constant source of energy and inspiration.

In March of 1998, many of those same people gathered in two churches over two evenings to sing together and celebrate Erin and our family. The purpose was to raise money for our trip to Salt Lake but the end result was priceless. Never had I ever felt more love and support than on that weekend. We were with friends and family who completely accepted who we were and I was singing! It was a beautiful weekend. Over four thousand dollars was raised. So many people gave freely of their time to make it a success.

So off we flew to Utah. These edited exerpts from my journal during the conference best describe the experience:

June 24 *— Here we are on the last leg of our journey to a new reality—at least this next new reality! I've been so nervous about this trip but now that we're almost there I feel a decided calm... underneath all the excitement! Up until now, I've been able to believe whatever I wanted.*

My imagination was the reality. In just a few hours, that will all change!

I won't be able to just make up the answers based on my own logic. I will be meeting many people who will actually define the new reality of not just the future, but who Erin is now and was these last five years. We will be able to talk about a new "norm".... something that I've always longed for. Yet, I'm not willing to do that now. I'm afraid that I will place limits on Erin, something I think I've avoided this far. After I meet these children who are older that Erin, will I ever be able to say, "Erin will be able to do anything, she'll just need time." ? I'm just coming to terms with the academic reality (almost)—-what if the physical is more than I can bear?! I know the truth is always the best and if I'm unprepared for the future, it will be harder to help Erin grow. But the old reality had become almost comfortable, or at least familiar.

June 25 — *This is so amazing! It is as overwhelming as I expected and there is a wealth of new information to wade through and decisions to make but it is very stimulating and satisfying. Whitney has been the highlight of our visit. At eleven and a half, she is exactly what we see Erin becoming. She is walking, talking, reading, friendly, helpful, outgoing ... and has the same facial expressions, mannerisms, posture as Erin. She even has a cousin Martha who gives her hand-me-down clothing, too! If Whitney is what Erin will grow up to be, I can handle that. It's not exactly what I pictured, but it is something I can handle. But most important, I can still believe it when I say: Erin will do whatever Erin will do ... at her own rate.*

The nice thing about this conference is I feel I could go to any of these people's homes and fit right in. We are all connected on some level that I haven't been able to identify. It's not looks and it's not just experience. It's more basic than that. Perhaps the geneticists are right and we are all related!

June 29 — *I actually had to figure out what day it is! What a great feeling. I've lived a lifetime in these past six days. The Hall's. The Sipes. Debbie and "Fridge"... and Tyson! The Shipps. The Fords. The list continues. Each has* *played a significant role in my functioning more effectively as Erin's parent. Deb said last night that she feels more empowered... and I agree. I am not the only one trying to do too many jobs, or on drugs to keep my stress from killing me. This conference has renewed my focus to help Erin learn. She has come so far, the doctors are very impressed with her. They feel she is in the top twenty-five percent and she scored well on her evaluative measures. They feel that she is unaffected by other complications and see a bright, positive future for her. We discussed tests to monitor kidney and retinal functions which can develop in JS kids over time.*

The memories of the conference fade too quickly as I sort through the things I said and saw to recall their impact:

- *bouncing Will and singing the Tigger song together with Erin*
- *seeing Timmy playing with Tyson and other "normal boys" his age.*
- *having a picnic with Whitney and hearing her confirm my suspicions of frustrations over language—-knowing what you want to say but not getting your mouth to say it.*
- *the realization that when Erin seems frustrated, I can give her concrete examples of who else feels that way and that in time, she can call, write or e-mail to share those frustrations with her peers.*
- *feeling a sense of family and connection with all those in the room*
- *seeing the tears in Milt's eyes when he shares his story*
- *appreciating the endless dedication of a few for the good of so many*
- *spending a beautiful day with the Sipes—rocks, photography, God and our children are common interests for us.*

The greatest impact on Erin's future from the conference was Bonnie Hanschu. Bonnie is part of Developmental Concepts in Arizona and developed a sensory processing therapy called The Ready Approach. A very intelligent woman with an "earth-mother" approach, Bonnie explains how Autism and Attention Deficit Disorder are sensory processing issues. She includes many examples of behaviours that are a direct result of sensory problems. We felt as if she was describing Erin! Erin had been having after school meltdowns, problems on car trips and first thing in the morning tantrums for a few years and they had been escalating. Bonnie talked about how the brain processes the environment and the neurochemicals involved. She also shared many stories of what a child with a sensory processing problem behaves like.

Kevin and I were so convinced that Erin's behaviours were sensory based, we made arrangements for me to fly to Seattle, WA to be trained in Sensory Processing therapy. We had been struggling with Erin for many months prior to our Salt Lake trip and had tried many techniques, mostly behaviour modification and "traditional" discipline. At certain times of the day and under certain circumstances, Erin would become enraged. It was never obvious what set her off and it is only with hindsight that I can pinpoint a pattern in the times and place. At the time we were living it, the behaviours seemed to be constant. Her behaviours would begin with her having problems asking for what she wanted. She would request something specific but when we gave it to her, she would shake her head no and ask for it again. Sometimes, she would just get stuck on a phrase and say it over and over getting angrier at every repetition. (I learned this is called perseveration: a characteristic commonly associated with autism in which the brain gets "stuck" and can't move on to the next thought.) As her anger escalated, she would begin hitting out around her: walls, floors, car windows, people—whatever she could reach. By this time, we would have removed her from the room the family was in, saying "we see you are angry but you are not allowed to behave this way. Come back when you have calmed down." She would come back calmer but usually escalated again within minutes. This would last anywhere from one to three hours. Kevin and I took turns being the parent and tried to be as consistent as possible but I must admit that after three hours our responses to her behaviour became a spanking with a teeth grinding "go to your room and stay there until we come to get you!" And since she couldn't open doors yet, if we closed it, she stayed in.

One day during a particularly difficult supper, Erin came back to the kitchen, tears streaming down her face saying she was sorry and she wouldn't hit any more. And all the while, her right arm was smashing against the dishwasher to the rhythm of her anger. It was at that moment that I suspected she could not control these "behaviours" and we needed help.

The more I learn about sensory processing the better I understand Erin. I had already decided that Erin's behaviours were not cognitively-driven; otherwise the behaviour modification techniques would have been more effective. The Ready Approach views behaviours as also neurochemically-driven. Depending on the "neuro-soup" being concocted in your brain , you will behave in different ways. If you have an elevated amount of dopamine, you could be aggressive or phobic (that innate fight/fright/flight response). A large amount of serotonin will elicit feelings of euphoria and well being (runner's high).

Since Erin was missing the vermis (a section which gates the information in and out of the cerebellum where the information is processed), her world was very confusing. [see Appendix B] Picture a horse race without a starting gate, some of the horses are facing the wrong way... and some aren't even on the track! The more input/output needed, the harder the job was:

talking — multiple muscles and thoughts to coordinate
walking — muscular and spatial
eating — a complete sensory experience (then add the noise and added smells of a restaurant? No wonder many kids "act up" in restaurants!)

All this confusion set up an increased dopamine response and because this neurochemical would spike so high, norepinephrine would also kick in to attend to the reason behind the increase. Simply put, Erin would go into sensory overload (more dopamine leading to aggressive behaviour) then her brain would focus on the overload and get stuck on trying to figure it out (perseveration and more aggression). For more information, visit Karen's website *www.brainjuice.ca*.

Well that's all nice in theory and the research looked sound (although many neurologists and doctors would say there was no real research) but what do I DO about it? By increasing the serotonin in your system, the neurochemicals regain an equilibrium and the brain can go back to its normal job and stop worrying about itself. So,

I learned about the Wilbarger brushing protocol; vestibular swings; proprioceptive input; focusing, calming and alerting activities; sensory diets; and on and on. [see Appendix C]

I came home from Seattle, walked in the house and began Erin's new therapy. Within the week, the behaviours decreased significantly. Within two months her speech had improved noticeably. Six months later, she was using a walker at school.

There are many other reasons for dramatic "growth spurts" in terms of gaining new skills in a child with neurological problems. The brain matures to a point which makes a whole group of milestones suddenly attainable (think of all the things you couldn't do if your brain lost contact with half of your tongue muscles). I believe that anytime you make a change in your routine, you see a change in behaviour. We had tried many other things over the years to assist Erin's development: chiropractor, allergens, natural healer, neutraceuticals, etc. All had elicited a short term change. But no other intervention has been so dramatic or long lasting. At the time of printing, we had been using the Ready Approach for two years and it still is able to help Erin manage her environment more effectively. She still has behaviours, but they never last more than twenty minutes and they are more predictable. Many kids with Joubert Syndrome use medications to control their aggressive behaviours and we may choose that route for Erin in the future. But for now, the natural serotonin enhancing therapies we administer are enough to maintain her equilibrium.

There have been many events in the past two years that have led Kevin and me to believe that the sensory processing therapy has been a major catalyst in the changes and growth that Erin has experienced. One benchmark was the sleep study we had done in the summer of 1999, which is where the writing of this story started. Despite all the equipment that the technicians in hospital scrubs hooked up to her, she never "lost it". The last two times we had been there, Erin was extremely uncomfortable when the lead lines were put on and seemed very afraid to move. She just lay on the bed with tears in her eyes until she finally fell asleep. This year, she was hesitant but cooperative and moved about freely on the bed until sleep overtook her. The results of the study were encouraging as well. This year, there were only 4.2 minutes per hour that she suffered apnea. I realize that within that year her brain had matured, she was farther away from the obstructive apnea that had been such a severe problem for her, and there were possibly other variables that I haven't even considered (environmental, etc.). But I also know, even though I can't isolate the effects to prove it, that the sensory therapy has made a significant difference for my daughter.

Erin's First Days

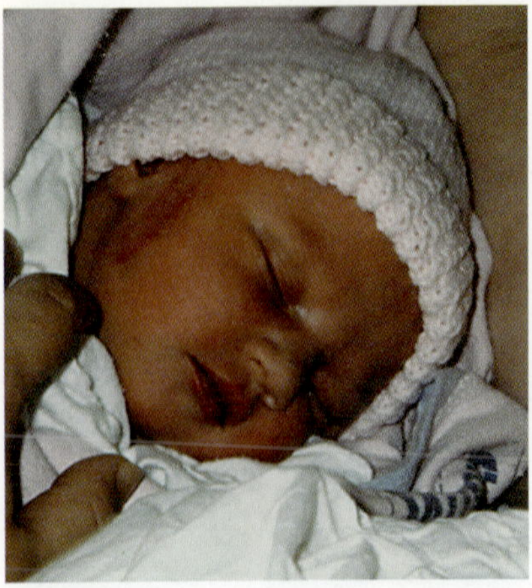

At fourteen hours

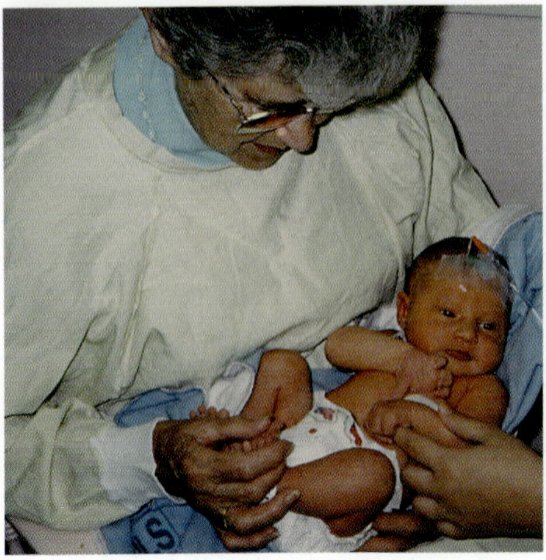

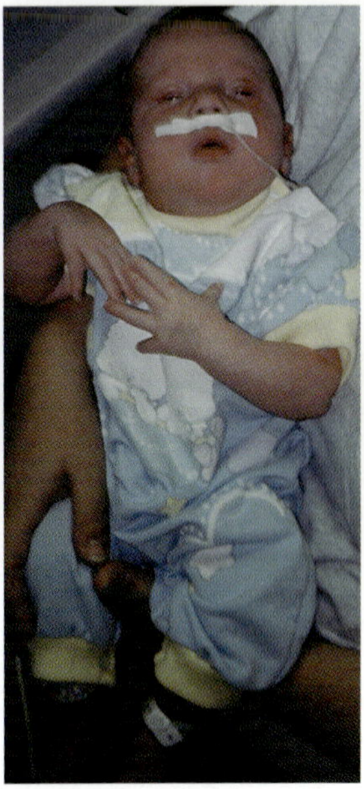

At four days *(above)*
with Grandma Bouw

At two and a half weeks *(right)*

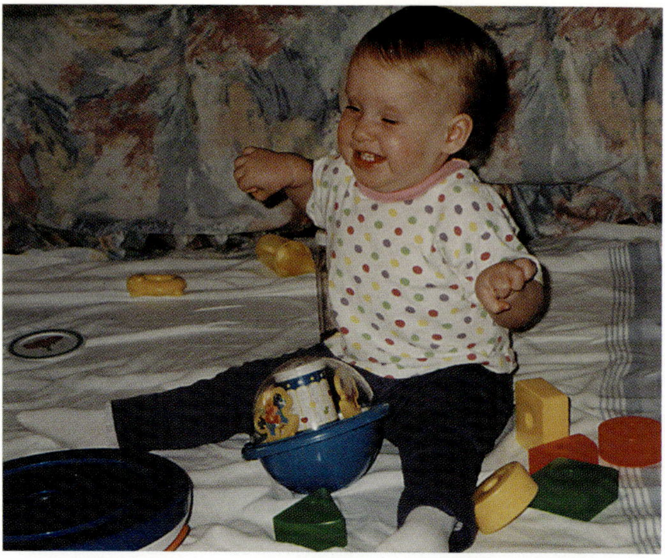

At fourteen months. Note the posture: "dinner-fork" arms, raised shoulders, and pointed toes.

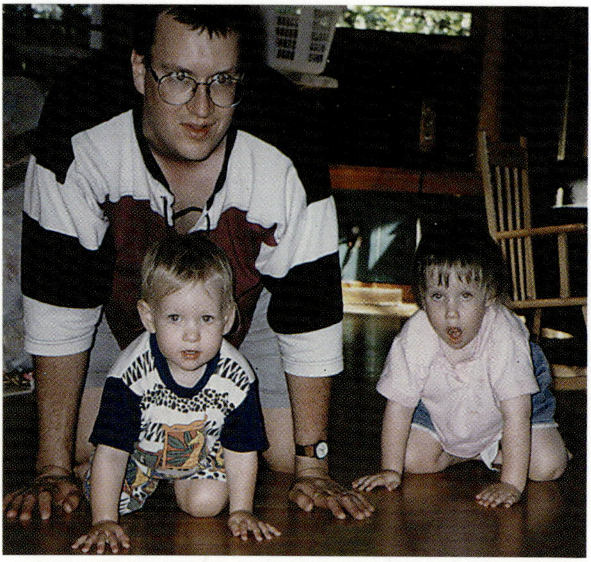

At two years. Playing zoo animals with Daddy and Sarah to learn to crawl.

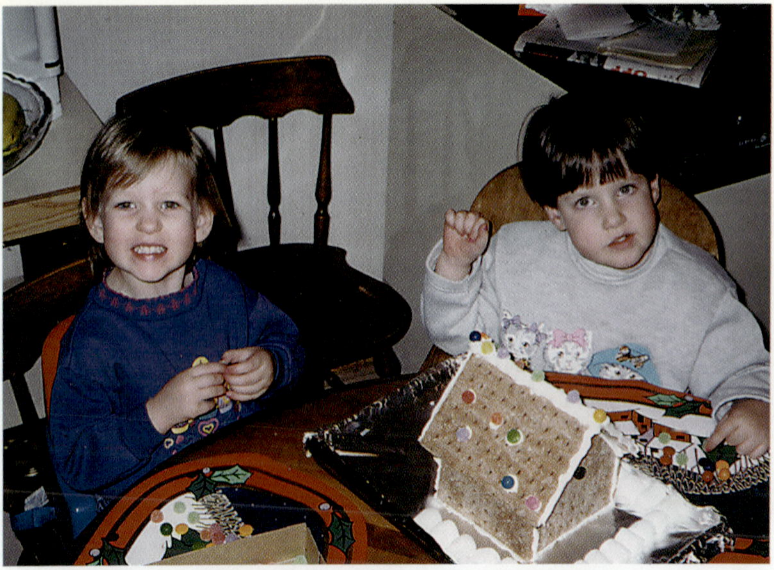

Gingerbread decorating is fun for fine motor.

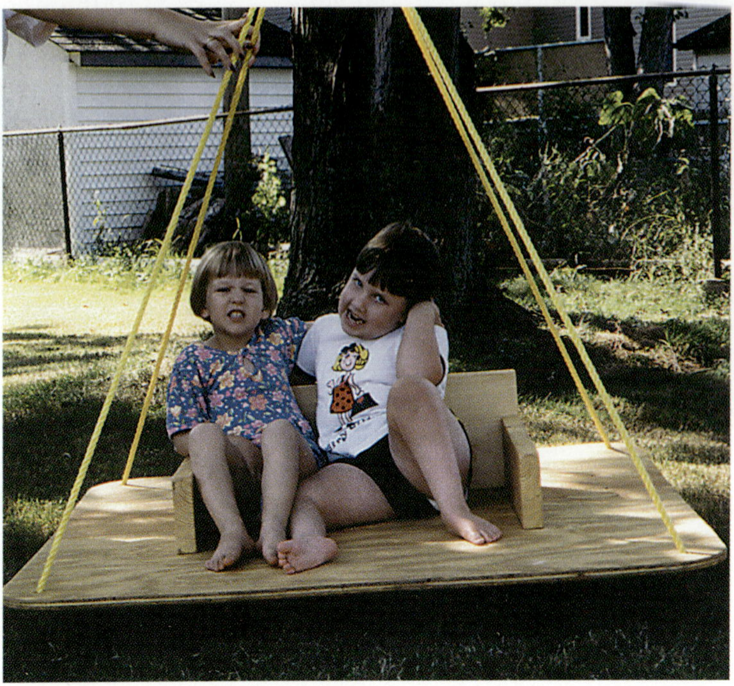

A vestibular swing is a must for sensory processing therapy

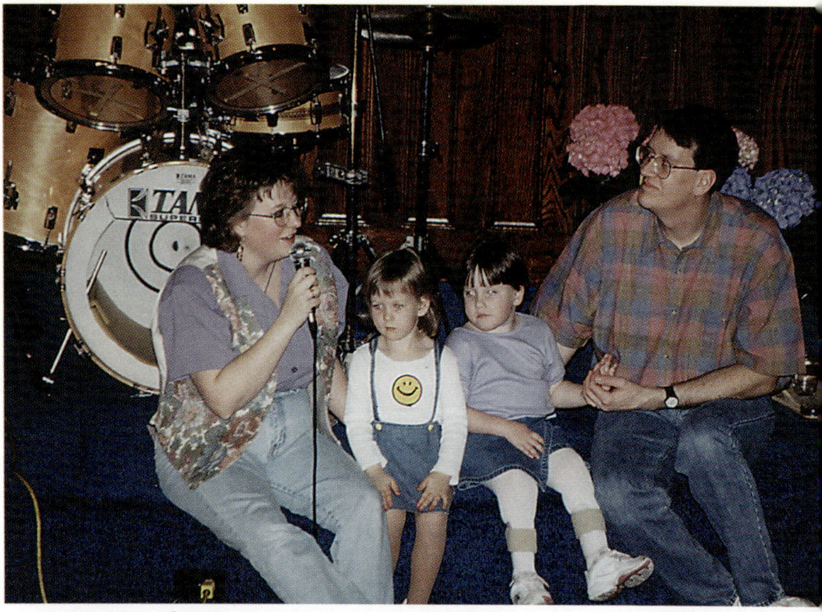

Music of Dreams was a community fundraiser to bring Erin to our first Joubert Syndrome Conference.

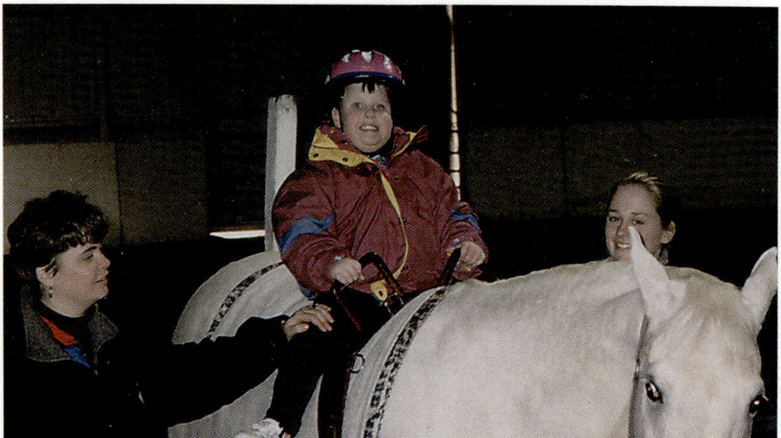

Hippotherapy is strongly recommended for many kids with special needs

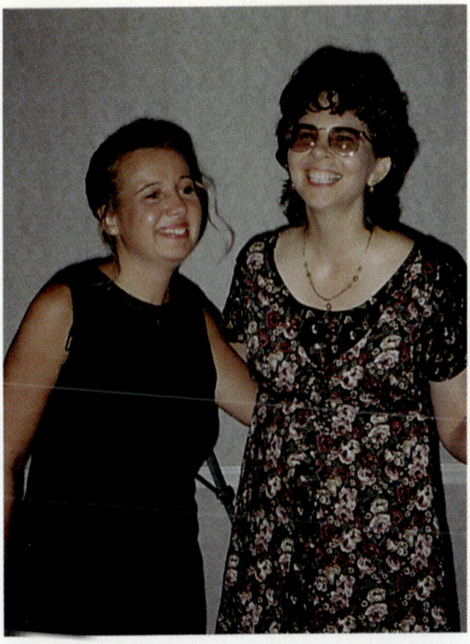

Cheryl Duquette (left), Mary Van Damme and Joanne Eastman (not shown) are the reason this book exists. Without their efforts in forming the Joubert Syndrome Foundation, Erin would not be where she is today.

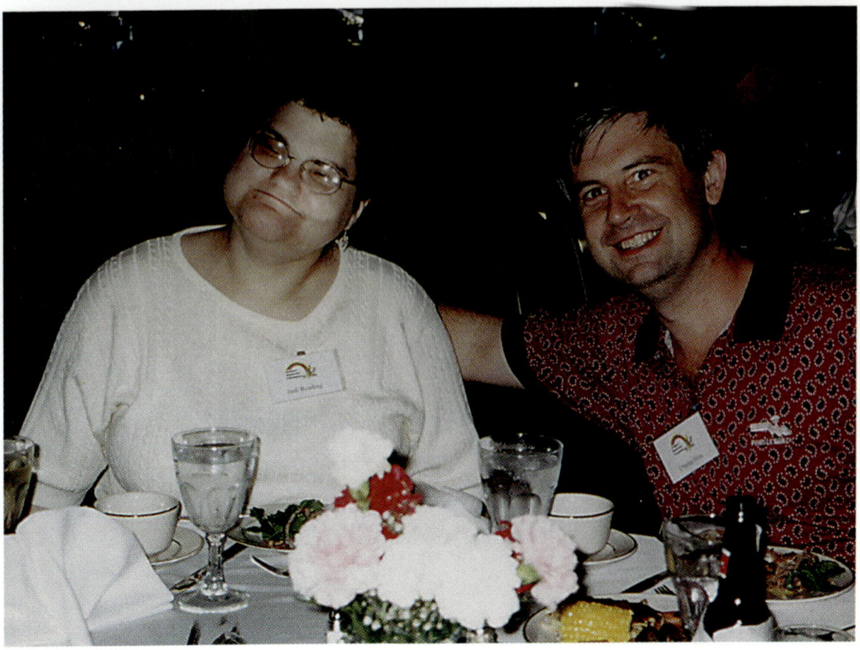

Judi and Charles at dinner at the Baltimore 2000 conference

Our Kids Love to Play

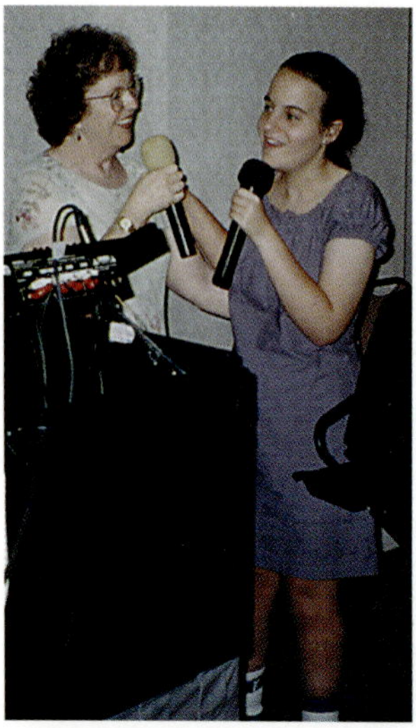

Stephanie (right) loves karaoke

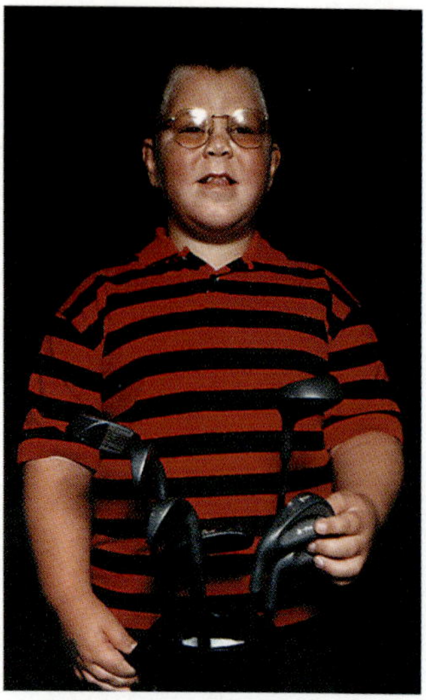

Ryan enjoys golf

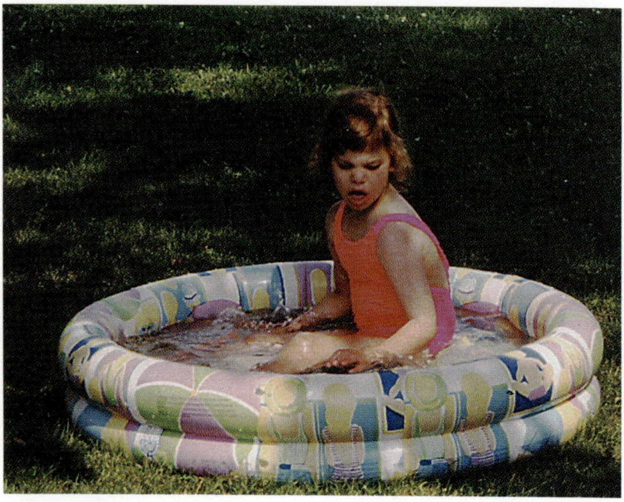

Alyssa likes the water

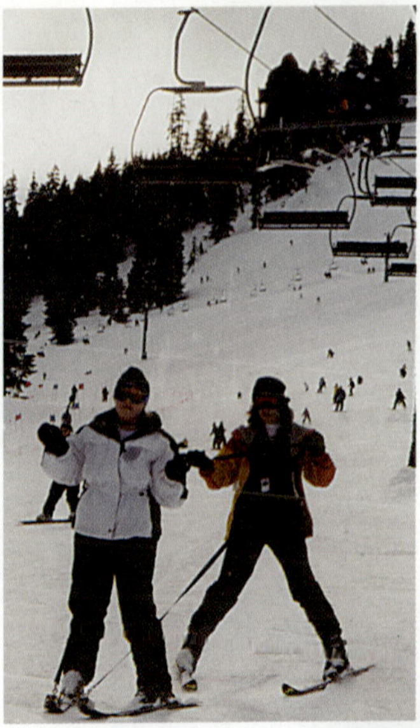

Whitney (left) on the slopes.

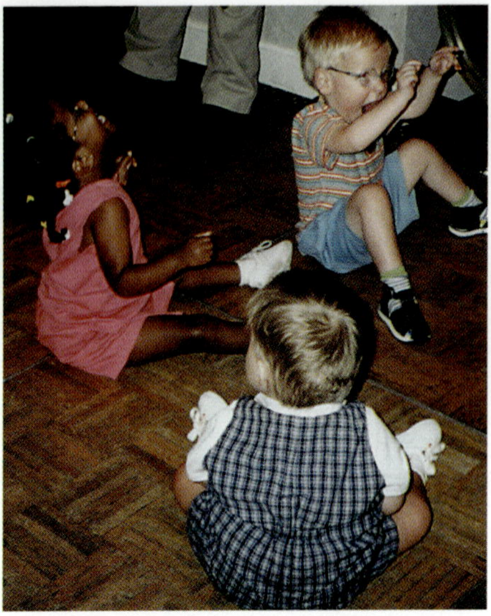

Taylor and George show their new friend the "bum scooch boogie"!

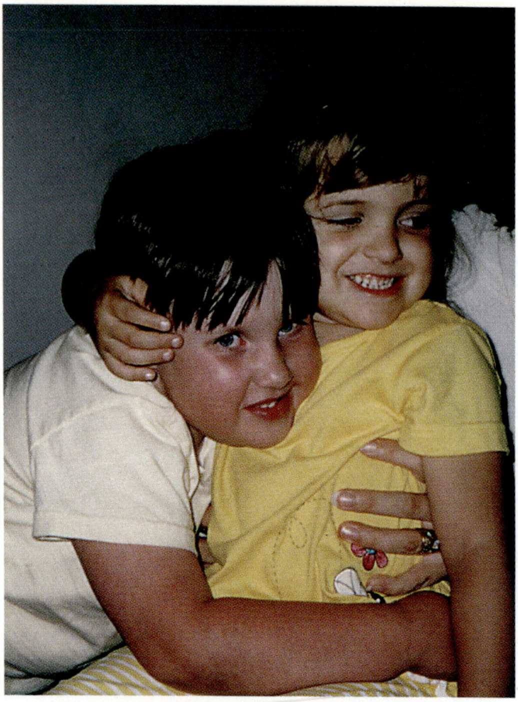

Lauren meets Erin in Niagara falls

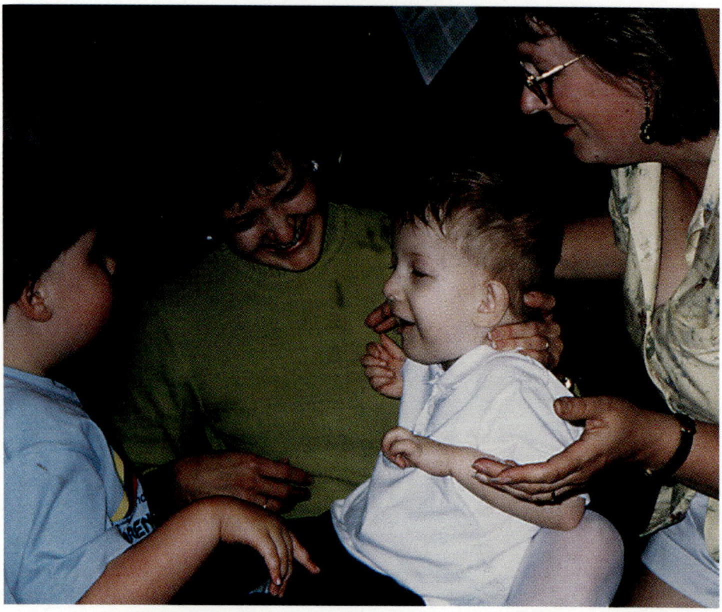

Will learns sign language at the Salt Lake City conference in 1998.

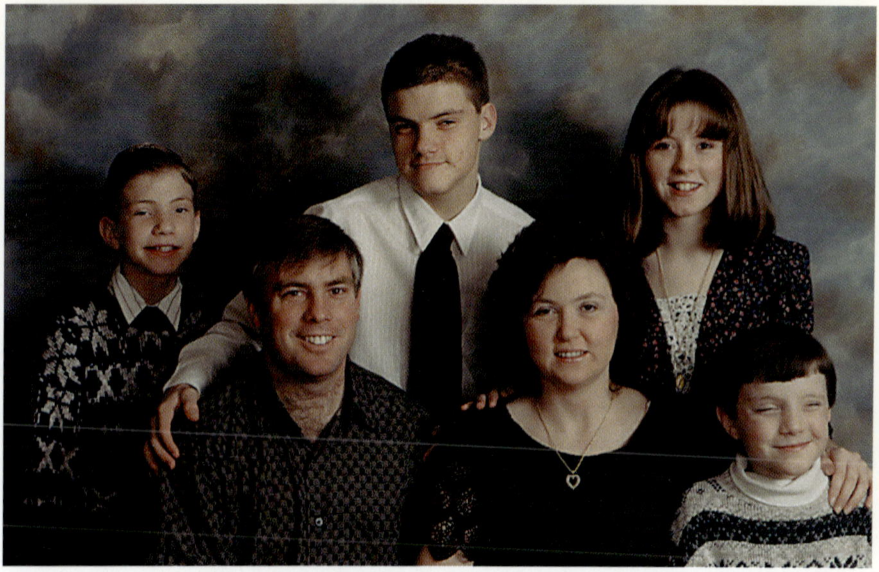

Sharie and family

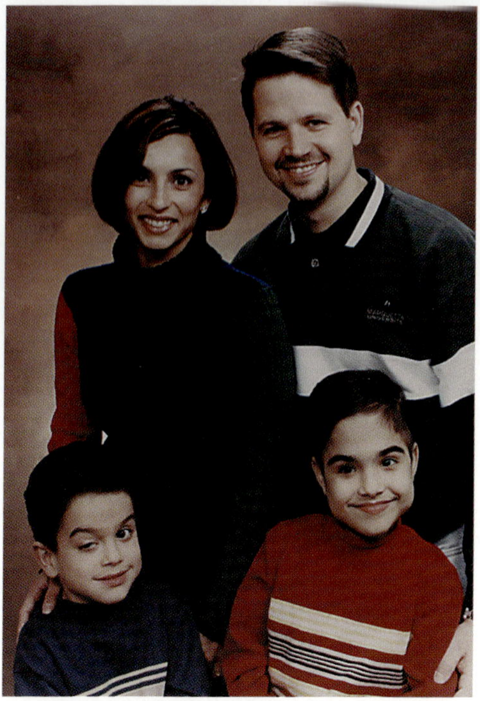

Jimmy and Jake with their parents.

... and Laugh

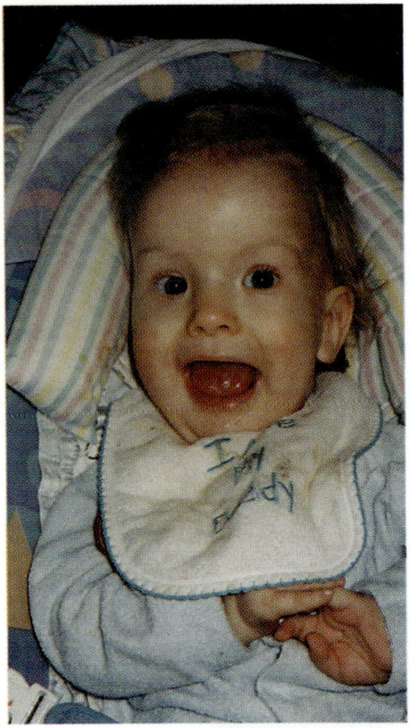

Aaron

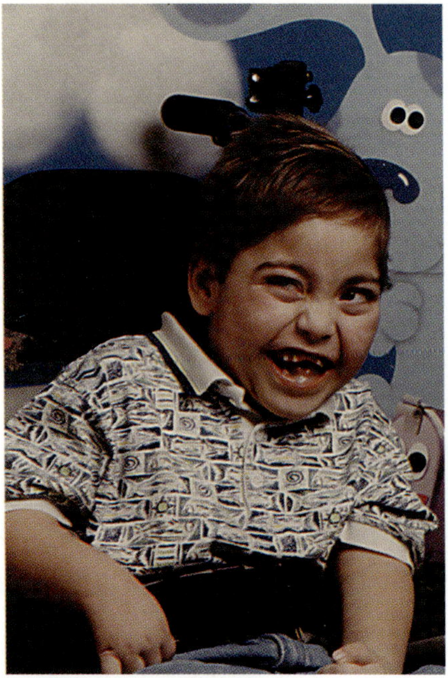

Joey

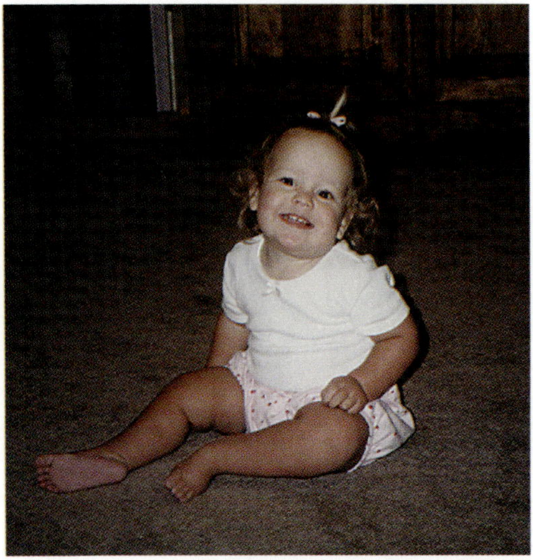

Caroline

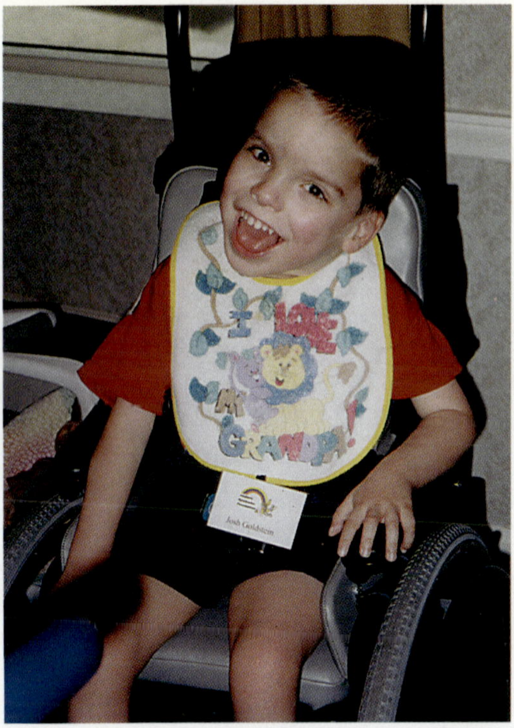

Josh

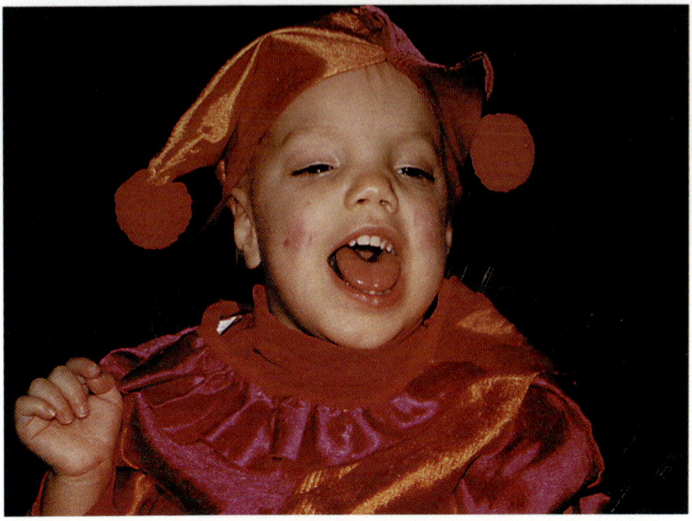

Abby ready for Halloween

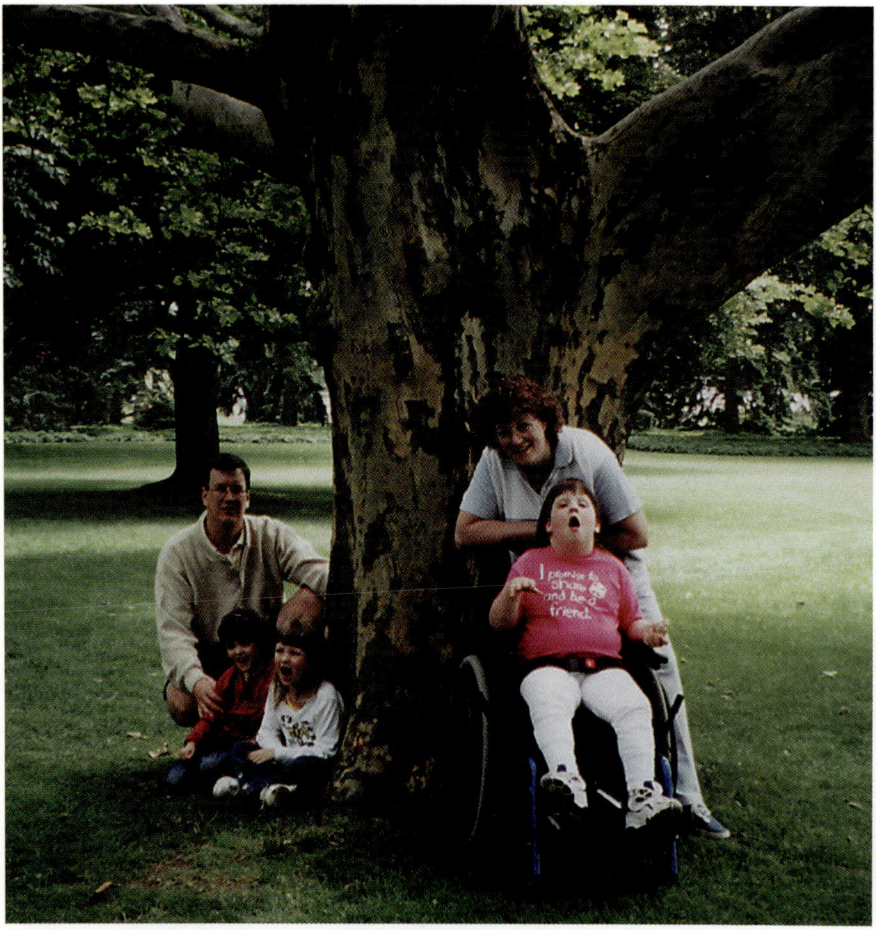

The Tompkins family:
Kevin, Heather, Sarah,
Karen, and Erin

Part Two

Other Stories

Alyssa

**excerpts from an article by Debbie Rose for* The Daily Press*: Escanaba, MI which appeared Saturday, January 16, 1993.*

Alyssa VanDamme is missing part of her brain.

The 2-year-old daughter of Mary and Tony Van Damme of Rock, Michigan has Joubert syndrome, a rare genetic disorder. It's estimated that about 10 cases occur each year in the United States, according to the National Organization for Rare Disorders. (NORD).

Alyssa was diagnosed with Joubert syndrome when she was 3½ months old.

After Alyssa was born Dec.12, 1990, she didn't open her eyes for almost two weeks, and when she would open them, they were only slits. Christmas Eve was the first time she opened her eyes for any length of time, Mary said.

The Van Dammes made an appointment with their family doctor to discuss Alyssa's eye problems. She referred them to a local opthamologist who suggested that Alyssa may be blind. She referred the Van Dammes to a neuro opthamologist [sic] and pediatric neurologist in Marshfield, Wis.

At the hospital in Marshfield, doctors ran a variety of tests—including magnetic resonance imaging (MRI)—on Alyssa on a Friday.

The Van Dammes had to wait the whole weekend for the results. The diagnosis: their daughter had Joubert syndrome.

"Supposedly it's pretty rare and it was identified as an entity in 1969," Mary said, adding that the neurologist hadn't seen a case of Joubert syndrome in his 15 years at the Marshfield hospital.

Alyssa is missing the vermis, which is part of the brain's cerebellum (the connecting tissue between the left and right hemisphere of the brain). The vermis controls coordination and balance.

The brain stem of Joubert syndrome children also is affected, causing abnormal eye movements and breathing abnormalities.

Mary says she had no physical complications or problems while pregnant for Alyssa.

"It was a normal pregnancy, and most are with this disorder," she said.

Since learning of Alyssa's condition, Mary has read all information she can find on Joubert syndrome. The prognosis does not look good.

Almost all literature she has read says Joubert children grow up severely, profoundly mentally retarded. According to the articles, she said, half die before the age of 5.

"I thought, 'Oh my God, this is awful.' I wanted to find other parents with kids who were affected to see if their kids were as seriously affected by it."

She then wrote to NORD and asked for a listing of parents who had children with Joubert syndrome.

Through the list, Mary made contact with six parents who had children with Joubert syndrome. Eventually, she and these parents formed a support group: Joubert Syndrome Parents-In-Touch Network. Whey the began the group last January, they had 8 parents and 10 children....

"We rely on each other because the doctors don't know that much about it, but parents who have experienced it will know."

Through the network, Mary has found some hope. Most parents of Joubert children she has talked to say their children are not severely mentally retarded. Some may be mildly retarded or moderately retarded. Some are of average intelligence and others are learning-disabled, she said.

A reason Joubert children may be classified as retarded, Mary believes, is because most aren't able to learn to coordinate their breathing and tongue movements because the vermis is missing. In the past, Mary said, it was assumed if one couldn't learn to speak, one couldn't learn and must be mentally retarded.

"They can't communicate and talk the way we do, but they had a lot upstairs," she contends.

Mary is hoping the network will be able to see that all children with Joubert syndrome are not automatically classified as severely retarded.

In some cases, parents are using picture communication cards and sign language to communicate with these children. Eventually, they may learn to communicate through computers, she said.

It is believed that these forms of communication can help alleviate the frustration that leads to self-mutilation, a common problem in Joubert children.

Mary and Tony have concerns about Alyssa's future and whether she'll ever be able to live independently. But they never question the love they have for her.

"She is an absolute joy to us and a very happy little girl and we wouldn't exchange her for anything."

Charles

I am not sure all the accolades should go to one particular person. My parents are two wonderful people who raised my brother and me the best way they could. My experiences in school were superb for the most part and I was lucky enough to have ingrained in me a strong sense of self.

My name is Charles Hine and I was born a decade before anyone had heard of Joubert Syndrome. The only diagnosis that made sense to the doctors was Cerebral Palsy so thus I began my journey. There were years of monotonous physical and speech therapy but I persevered. Nothing would get the better of me and I would prevail! Being stubborn can work for you sometimes and I was the epitome of stubbornness. Of course, if one wants to move mountains, one has to have some willingness to be uncompromising in that pursuit of "perfection". From an early age I was with my peers in a "regular" classroom setting. My parents had a lot to do with this and hence my stubborn streak. Mainstreaming was certainly not a common way of educating students with disabilities back in the 60's. My parents, therefore, must have run into obstacles along the way but I never (well...hardly ever) felt segregated from my peers. For the most part, I've had good experiences but of course if a child has a wider gait than his or her other peers, or the speech patterns are unique then finger-pointing and jeering are almost guaranteed on some occasions. Children and adults can be afraid to approach or strike up a conversation with anyone who appears to be different but you go on and I was stubborn enough to move my life forward. Ignoring rude remarks was my defense mechanism and I tried hard to ignore those remarks. Sometimes I just could not let bygones be bygones though so I got to know the inside of the principal's office too. Many of my teachers were patient and very nurturing; almost as much, and I have to say sometimes more so, than my parents.

If there's one thing I've learned from life so far, it is that children grow in direct proportion to the love and support given to them by the significant adults in their life. Encouragement to repeat good deeds and attain goals (however small) will go a long way in developing an adult with the confidence and, dare I say, stubbornness to succeed in life. The way my parents raised me obviously worked for me; support/encouragement tempered with a dose of reprimand for negative behavior. One can not necessarily expect a well-adjusted and emotionally healthy adult if that adult was not held accountable for unhealthy behavior as a child. It was thus my responsibility (I say that now) to do what my parents told me or suffer the consequences.

Let me skip ahead to more recent events. These included attending college (1981–1985) where I obtained a degree in English and Communications, and graduate school (1983–1985) where I earned my Masters in Social Work. By the time I entered college, I was feeling pretty good about myself and my ability to succeed on my own. This confidence came primarily from my parents' decision to enroll me in a small, private high school that emphasized personal attention and put the onus on the student to learn at his or her own pace. This kind of educational setting forced those students who were serious about the learning process to flourish. I was motivated so when college rolled around I was ready to jump in with both feet. The college I decided to attend was very small in terms of student enrollment but really spread out in terms of area. This being the case, I made sure that any back-to-back classes were both on the "north" or "south" campus. There were also services for students with disabilities such as copying material in the school library and early registration to avoid long lines. These services certainly made my higher education less taxing and a lot more enjoyable.

The love and support I've received from many people has been a key ingredient in what I have become today. The child growing up with Joubert Syndrome, or any disability for that matter, could benefit greatly from being treated like any other child. Apart from medical considerations such as seizures, negative behaviors need to be dealt with just as any other child growing up without a disability. All families and children are unique so my experiences won't necessarily reflect any one else's. What I can tell others though is that I responded favorably to people who encouraged me to build on what I could do. Also, instill some stubbornness in your children to succeed. In my opinion, that can't be bad.

Charles and William

by "Mom" 8/93

Charles and William are of a generation before CT scans and MRI's, therefore they have never had an official medical diagnosis of Joubert Syndrome. However, having become aware of Joubert Syndrome in the past year through the amazing efforts of Mary Van Damme, Cheryl Duquette and JoAnne Eastwood and my work at the Connecticut Parent Advocacy Center, (a member of the National Network of Parent Training and Information Centers funded through the U.S. Dept. of Education) we feel convinced that they had and continue to exhibit a number of the symptoms of JS as documented in the papers we have read. Having also talked with Dr. D (one of a very few pediatric geneticists working on Joubert Syndrome) at the recent Joubert Syndrome Parents-In-Touch Network Conference in Washington, and having met there so many children who appear to be so similar to Charles and William at the same age, we are even more convinced that this offers an explanation of their disorder. We had never encountered any children before that we could say "just like our boys"!

Both boys were given, and we accepted, an initial diagnosis of "ataxic cerebral palsy". However they never seemed to fit this diagnosis or develop as most children with CP that we knew. In fact one person who worked closely with them and other children with cerebral palsy throughout the country once commented that she had never encountered any child with such severe ataxia as Charles and William exhibited. At the age of about 18 years after a CT scan William was determined to have "cerebellar dysgenesis," and we have used that diagnosis for them since because it seemed more precise to describe their disability. We do not have that information about Charles but both boys are similarly involved.

Charles was born in December 1958 and William was born in June 1960 after normal, uneventful and full-term pregnancies. Almost immediately after birth Charles developed rapid breathing (180 a minute) and was placed in an oxygen tent for three days. The breathing stabilized and he and I went home on the fourth day. He was a difficult baby, very wakeful, impossible to console, startled easily, had a difficult time sucking, cried a lot—but was healthy and beautiful with seemingly normal development. However at 4 months I noticed his eyes did not track and that they "crossed" a lot. Many of my maternal observations were put on record as "first baby syndrome"! By a year old he definitely had pronounced strabismus, he could manage to roll over and if placed in a sitting position could maintain it momentarily with some support. He was excessively hypotonic with no trunk control and "jelly legs." His mouth was lax and he drooled constantly. I was able to carry him in a portable "Infanseat" until he was too big to fit into it. He could not raise himself from the angled position, he was like a rag doll. By 18 months he could get to a sitting position himself and could pull himself to a standing position in a net playpen, but could grasp the rail very briefly before falling. He had no balance and no real motor coordination nor reflexes to break his fall. He was a bright and responsive child, but with no signs of speech. By the age of two he could maneuver himself around in a walker with a sling body support. He could not crawl but could drag himself with his arms on his belly. This was his means of independent travel for the next few years until he could grasp furniture to keep his balance in an upright position. We encouraged normal walking by supporting him from behind holding both hands for balance and support, and he "strutted" using alternate legs.

He had a tremor and fine motor skills were a real problem. Startle reflexes were exaggerated throughout childhood. By the age of three and a half he could put two words together but words had no endings and were single syllables. He had corrective eye surgery at the age of three years after we moved to Connecticut. He attended a preschool program for children with cerebral palsy from age two years nine months and we began physical, occupational and speech therapy. He was evaluated by Dr. A in 1962 (The attending pediatrician after his birth had an interest in genetics and worked closely with Dr. A), by a number of orthopedic specialists at a children's hospital here in Connecticut, and at the rehabilitation center in New Hampshire in 1963 before entering kindergarten. Several educational evaluations were used as guidance through his school years. Medical evaluations always ruled out most likely causes or diseases or conditions and gave us a "probably genetic" result, without anything definitive. The problem was intriguing to the medical personnel but unfathomable.

Although initial evaluations had given him an IQ of 74, after the workup at the center they suggested he had an IQ closer to 120! They recommended that he be placed in first grade rather than kindergarten because of the less physical activities involved. He entered regular first grade in the local school in a wheelchair, and spent two years in first grade and then progressed normally through elementary and middle school with some adaptations such as a typewriter and peer assistance. There was a lot of watching from the sidelines I am afraid. Always present but not always included, although everyone tried hard. However most of his interests and activities followed the interests and activities of his contemporary age group.

During a residential stay at the rehabilitation center he

was equipped with crutches and taught how to use them with a four point gait. He was not secure with crutches until about the age of seven. He continued therapy throughout his grade school years and was closely followed by orthopedists at the children's hospital. We were introduced to the Bobath method of therapy (Neuro-developmental Training) on visits to grandparents in England and encouraged its use by therapists here. It helped a lot with balance stimulation. Speech was by now intelligible but tongue manipulation was a problem and speech therapy concentrated on repetitive exercises to teach him tongue control and placement.

He attended a regular private high school that allowed him to progress at his own rate, and he was by then able to ambulate with just a cane for balance. He graduated from high school and entered a four year state college, where he majored in English with a minor in Communication. He graduated in 1979. He now walks without supports but has a "drunken" gait. He has hesitant speech albeit articulate and clear. Less able fine motor skills still interfere, but he enjoys playing golf! Charles returned to school two years after receiving his Bachelor's degree because he could not find appropriate employment and he received a Master's degree in Social Work from the University of Connecticut in 1983. He has lived independently since entering graduate school and is able to support himself. He is able with computers, writes well and has a good work ethic, but has not been successful in finding a really satisfying career field.

William's entry into the world was different. He had no breathing problems at birth and all seemed well, until he too developed a severe strabismus and could just hold his head up at five months old, and from that point his development was identical to that of Charles. The same lax, open and drooling mouth, the same hypotonia, and "jelly" legs, even greater startle reflex, but the same engaging and responsive personality. William had corrective eye surgery at the age of two and a half, which was not quite as successful as Charles' surgery and he had "tracking" problems that persist, but do not interfere at this stage.

We returned to Dr. A's when William was about 19 months old in 1962 to enable him to do further testing as part of his chromosome studies. He also saw Charles at that time as an outpatient, but William was studied for about a month as an inpatient. At this time most known disorders were ruled out and Dr. A gave a "catch-all" diagnosis of cerebral palsy for want of some description of the presenting symptoms. He determined that the origin was "probably genetic" and stated that one certain factor was that he was probably an intelligent child because he was so persistent. He based this observation on the fact that William was constantly pulling himself to standing in the crib and falling like a log as soon as he grasped the rail, only to get right back up again - just as Charles had done.

So William joined Charles in the same therapy sessions (generally back-to-back) and in the educational journey two years behind his brother who paved the way with the educators. William also attended regular classes in the local elementary and middle schools with resource room help for English and Math when needed, and then the same private high school that Charles was at. William had more of a tremor and a greater balance problem than Charles, but his persistence and determination kept him pretty much abreast of his brother, physically. His speech was more severely affected, being very flat and monotonal. It created enormous frustration in his childhood and adolescence. His speech was virtually unintelligible to anyone except those familiar with his speech patterns - and even to those sometimes. Only in adulthood has he persevered and been able to develop good communication skills. Most people can understand his slow and persevering speech, but the disability is more evident than his brother's. He was also a slower learner than Charles and spent more time in the special education resource room with remedial help with math and writing. He too progressed from a wheelchair to crutches and a four point gait to a cane and now to an unsupported "drunken" gait. The exaggerated startle reflex has persisted and William still "jumps out of his skin" when he is startled by loud noises.

William did not go to college, but for the past eight years he has lived independently and has supported himself in full-time employment as a library technician in a government documents library in the city where he lives. He spends most of the rest of his life working with amateur theatrical groups, and following his lifelong interest in musical theater and monster movies and old-time radio. He has appeared on stage with a local group, volunteers his time with the local arts center and has a pretty good "quality of life."

Both boys participated in a therapeutic horseback riding program in their teen years that was an enormous benefit both for balance stimulation and their self confidence. Although Charles has allergies, especially hay fever, both boys have had good physical health as they have developed, the most frequent visits to the emergency room being to stitch up chins, or necks or hands suffered in "dead falls." It must be said that neither William nor Charles now drool—maternal persistence in repetitively chucking them under the chin trained them otherwise, and that symptom was eliminated by school age! We are very proud of them both and admire their determination to be the best that they can be in whatever they undertake.

Postscript:

Joubert Syndrome was first identified in 1969 and is a very rare genetic disorder due to a recessive gene that still has to be identified as the marker (the chromosome has been identified but there is a long way to go from there!) It has to be present in both parents and could well be present in many others (a 50/50 chance) in the extended families but they just haven't met another with the same gene. Even if they have done so, the children need not necessarily be affected: witness our son Jack! And another family in Utah had five syndrome-free children before their sixth child was almost a duplicate of our William!

The symptoms vary but almost all children exhibit breathing difficulties at or soon after birth, severe startle reflexes, and eye problems, hypotonia, and fine and gross motor and/or speech defects. Some children do have mental retardation or autistic behaviors, but most do not even though their responses may be slow. These symptoms are caused by the complete or partial absence of the cerebellar vermis that is only apparent in a CT scan or MRI.

So far approximately 175 or so families have been identified worldwide, although the number is growing, due greatly to the three mothers in Michigan, Virginia and Maryland who were put into contact with each other through Dr. D. They formed an international network of parents, the Joubert Syndrome Parents-In-Touch Network, to share information and support through a newsletter and a conference, to educate physicians and to increase public awareness and encourage research. In 1997 the name of the organization was changed to Joubert Syndrome Foundation to reflect its nonprofit status.

Robert

Robert was born at three o'clock on the afternoon of January 1st, 1966. The day was very warm and pleasant. The day and the weather conditions are very important to note because they represent Robert. He was a very warm and pleasant young man with a refreshing outlook on life. Robert was very reserved, kind and considerate. Robert enjoyed people and was always pleasant to be with. He knew that he did not have to be loud and rowdy to be a man. Robert never had to go to work or school on his birthday and he always told us so when he was wished a happy birthday at the close of the annual ARC New Years Eve party.

At age three, he attended preschool on Lilac Lane and at age four, he went to the State hospital for physical and speech therapy. He was moved back home after one and a half years. He went to local elementary and high schools graduating from a special education setting. After graduating, he was placed on a waiting list for an opening at Hillman, a local community support center.

During the time between graduation and going to the Center, Robert stayed at home alone and would read the newspaper from cover to cover. When asked what was in the paper, he would get the paper and show you where he had underlined the words he knew in the article he wanted to talk about, and then tell you what it said. Then he would show you the more interesting parts of the paper. He was always very accurate as to the content of the article and was always disturbed by tragic news. He always knew what was on TV and showing at the movies. During these times he grew in wisdom and understanding. When his brother was learning the multiplication tables Robert surprised us all by doing the same and would race to give the answers.

Robert started working at Hillman in 1986. He worked many jobs there and enjoyed most of them. He would always tell us what he worked on and how many pieces he'd completed. He really liked the job club and was always the first one there. Recently Robert was employed at Fast Serve Imaging Inc. along with working in the Hillman work shop. He looked forward to going to work at Fast Serve Imaging Inc. and riding the city bus. He was always excited about his pay checks and would enjoy taking them to the bank. He was teased about taking the family out to eat since he had so much money, but somehow the bill was always paid before he got the chance to pay it.

Robert attended the RNC (Religious Nurture Center) at the First United Methodist church for 25 years. He loved the RNC and would go to the Wednesday fun nights and other social get together. When he moved into the Hillman group home, he was instrumental in getting the group home to go to the RNC. He also would attend the Thursday Bible study class if he did not have square dancing with the Rocking Squares.

Robert and his family were members of the YMCA for years, and they spent many hot summer days swimming and playing at the pool. Robert made friends with all of the people that came to the pool and would play water games with them. Robert liked doing active things like riding the bike, bowling, swimming, tennis, basketball, hiking, and going for a two to three mile walk with his family.

Robert participated in many activities. Some of these were the special Olympics and ARC activities. Robert started with the Special Olympics from the dirt tracks in Winfield and grew with them over a period of 25 years as the Special Olympics grew to WSU. Robert's life represents the "if you can't win be brave, true and honest in the attempt" portion of the special Olympic oath. He stopped participating in the Special Olympics when his doctors told him he should find a different level of competition to participate in.

Robert enjoyed and had a special talent for music. He would practice his piano for hours and would play much of that time totally from memory. He also played at several Special Education workshops in an effort to demonstrate that he may have been mentally handicapped but given the chance he could rise above those limits with astounding ability. Robert also played the piano during several recitals at WSW. When working toward those recitals he was told that all of the others would have to play their piece from memory but he could use his music book. Well, that was not good enough for him so Robert memorized his music to the amazement of everyone and often received a standing ovation.

Robert liked to go on vacation. These vacations began early in his life and they took Robert and his family through the Midwest, Hawaii, and the Caribbean. Therefore, when it came to traveling with the ARC and Hillman, he was always ready to go. In fact he was packed a month ago to go on a vacation with his family next week.

On one of the family vacations, Robert and his brother Douglas were fishing when Robert caught a fish and hollered with excitement. A young girl turned to see what the excitement was about which put her in range of the fish that Robert was reeling in. So, as Robert jerked the fish out of the water, the fish struck the girl right in the mouth resulting in a scream from the girl. This was followed by a, "Robert, why did you let that girl kiss your fish?" comment from Doug and a hardy round of laughter from everyone around. Through the years any time Doug wanted to make Robert smile he would say something about "Rob was the only one that had girls kiss his fish" and Robert would get a big grin. Given a chance, Robert would be fishing. Some times he would out-fish his dad and would tease him about that.

Robert loved the fellowship of his family and friends. He liked to be teased and he got a lot of that from his dad and brother. But mostly he liked to be happy and to be with others who were happy. Robert liked animals and pets, especially Tootsie and Nikki the two family dogs.

Robert liked helping with fund raisers. One event Robert always looked forward to was assisting with the Charley Daniel Golf tournament. He also looked forward to meeting all of the performers who came to help Hillman. One of his favorite groups was Mason Dixon and specifically a special friend Caz who is a member of that group. Some of Robert's friends have made it possible for Caz to be here. Caz has traveled a great distance to be here today with his special friend and to personally represent their special friendship.

Robert liked concerts and would go when his parents or brother would take him. In the last few years he went to the Wranglers baseball games and was a ten year veteran fan of the Wichita Wings. He has a prized ball signed by all of the Wings players. His brother made these arrangements to ensure that the Wings knew they had at least one devoted fan. His room always contained several posters from sporting events that he attended.

Robert accepted all of the challenges in his life with total commitment. He would accept the opportunity to figure out how to make things work on the computer or quickly figure out how to make a VCR or tape player work so he could record special programs and spend hours making special music tapes that he would then share with his friends and family.

Robert liked to dance and was eager to learn how to do many of the new dances. He was an active square dancer and was a member of a square dance group. He liked all kinds of music especially music with soul such as gospel, country and western, the old time rock and roll, and some classics. He learned the Macarana and would perform it flawlessly. He taught it to everyone in his group home and Robert was always the hit of the dance with his innate musical ability. People would sit and watch him in amazement that he could dance so well. Robert had many friends, but he also had a special friend named Michelle. He liked to take her to the movies, dances, and just spend time with her.

Some times she would invite him over for a meal and

to watch TV with her and her roommate. Other times he would invite her over to his group home for the evening. Robert always wrote her a letter each day. In his last and unfinished letter to her, he asked her if she would like to hold his hand and go to the movies.

Robert liked all children, and would play and share things with them. He liked to help take care of babies, especially feed and rock them. Robert treated everyone as he wanted to be treated, that is, with fairness, kindness, and consideration. Robert made and treated everyone as a friend. He was known by many and was always admired by long time acquaintances as well as those who just met him.

Robert only got to spend a short time with the latest addition to his family but was very excited to welcome his-sister-in-law into it. He was always ready to do anything that involved Doug and Terri. There were many times that Robert would stick up for Terri when Doug would tease her and Terri would return the favor for Robert. Robert looked forward to assisting in Terri and Doug's wedding. He also looked forward to the wedding dance. Especially since Terri said that she and Robert would do the Macarana. Well, he woke that group up in his own style. When the first fast beat song was played Robert was in action and as usual he made smooth moves right with the beat. He enjoyed the dance but really lit up when it was time to do the Macarana with Terri. He talked about dancing with Terri and said, "Terri like to dance with me."

On Friday August 15, 1997 Robert was attending a swimming outing at Edgemore park swimming pool when something went wrong—we can only wonder what and why. Robert is now in God's loving arms. Robert is greatly missed by many. He has touched so many lives and put nothing but happiness into the lives of those that knew him. Especially his family and many friends.

Ben's Eulogy

By Ben's Mom

No more oxygen tanks, pulse oxymeters, and vile medications. No more standers and wheelchairs and AFOs. No more nebulizer treatments and cleaning vomit off the carpet. No more late night emergencies, hospitalizations, tubes, wires, and syringes. Blessed relief.

No more hugs and kisses. No more crooked smiles. No more delighted full-body wiggles. No more roughhousing on the floor. Wretched grief.

My son died. Some say there is no greater pain than to lose a child. I'm sure there are many here today who feel that pain every bit as keenly as I do. Ben touched many people very deeply. That pain would not hurt so much if the love was not so deep. There is no greater love than that of a parent for a child.

Benjamin was only 3 years old when he died. In three short years, Ben faced more medical problems than most people do in 75 years of life. He was hospitalized six times, rode the ambulance four times, and has taken many medications every day for the past 2 1/2 years in order to stay as healthy as possible. His disabilities and health impairments have hardly been conducive to a "normal" lifestyle. Life has been difficult for all of us these past three years - but I would not trade a second of it. Ben was an incredible gift of love and I am so grateful for the time I had with him.

Many years ago, I prayed for patience. So God sent me Meglyn, my first-born. And I learned. But I was still dissatisfied with my ability to cope with such an energetic child. So I prayed for more patience. And God sent me Madison. Between the two of them, I learned how to be patient with all kinds of children. But still I didn't think I was quite where I needed to be. So I prayed some more and God sent me Ben. That's when I learned how to be patient with adults, too.

Madison and Ben have both brought into my life such diversity and an understanding of the bigger picture. From the moment five years ago, when the ophthalmologist shook his head and said my daughter would never see, I knew life would never be the same. I was not allowed to stay the same, to become stagnant in my abilities and thinking. In advocating for their needs in the education, social service, and medical systems, I grew in every way. Meeting their needs has done more to help me purge selfishness and pettiness from my heart, and develop a deeper understanding and compassion for all people. My children have molded me to be confident in my ability to tackle the various hurdles we have faced in those arenas than any other experience I've ever had. Ben especially gave me the courage to face my worst fears and still do the best job I could as a mother.

Before I had children, I never would have guessed the depth of the love that a mother could feel. Meglyn taught me how deeply a mother can love. Madison taught me that I can love all children. Ben showed me how to love all people. He has taught me how to love completely and selflessly.

Ben has moved me to learn more, do more, be a better person than I was. Even though he was blind, he gave me eyes to see what I had not seen before. Even though he was deaf, he taught me to listen with an open heart and mind. Even though he was very sick, he gave me enormous strength.

Ben gave me such joy. The smallest things gave me the most enormous pleasures. The brief moments that I could hold his hand, the rare times he was able to hug back, the times he was able to let me hold him for hours at a time, and even roughhouse on the floor, the beautiful smiles, the stiff wiggle of his body when he was delighted.... These moments were better than vacations, promotions, and fancy parties. With his needs for expensive health care and equipment, I knew I'd never drip with diamonds—better, I dripped with joy and happiness.

Because of Ben, I have known complete joy and happiness. I thank God everyday for sending him to me.

I believe that Ben has fulfilled his purpose here on Earth. Many of us spend decades trying to do what we are called to do: invent something, improve something, whatever. Some never do fulfill their calling. In just three short years, Ben has done more; through him, souls are saved. Look around you—feel the love here. He has touched each of us deeply and we are forever changed.

To those of you who were afraid of his disability and health impairments, please let his life and death inspire you to reach out to others in need. To any who are afraid, feel the strength here and carry it out into the world with you. If you are lonely, take heart that it is in the giving of love to others that you learn to feel truly loved.

You have all been so kind to me in the past several days. The phone calls, cards, food, gifts, flowers, and words of love and encouragement have lifted my spirit and helped me endure the grief of the loss of my son. Thank you. I know you feel very sad for me. But it is that feeling, that ability to truly feel caring and giving, that inspires the best in all of us. Don't turn that off over the next few days. Let that pain turn into the glow of joy and the ability to easily give to anyone in need at any time. In that way, my loss is not in vain and Ben's life and death will have helped so many people. Thank you so much for being here with us today.

Whitney

Whitney has always been rather accepting of her disability—just accepting the fact that she is different, that her body and brain may not work quite like everyone else's but that's okay. I have to admit that we've worked real hard at helping her understand that it's okay to be different.

If you ask her now, she will tell you that she has Joubert Syndrome and that she has one kidney and perhaps even talk a little about her eyes, etc., then she'll start telling people about other kids who have Joubert (of course, this has been once we got the diagnosis of Joubert 2 years ago and then met the Totennellys—now she will start listing off just about every kid she met in Salt Lake City!).

One of the greatest stories took place probably when she was in second grade back in Iowa. She was working away in her special ed classroom and the principal came in with some guests (the special ed program in that school district had many accolades and thus a lot of folks came to visit). At any rate, Mr. S said, "This is our handicapped classroom." Whitney turned around at him and said very matter-of-factly, "I not handicapped. I special." Of course, that stopped him dead in his tracks but honestly I guess that's how Whitney has always viewed herself. When we didn't have diagnosis or easy words to describe her symptoms those first 9-10 years, we talked about how she was just special and that things others could do that would be harder for her or impossible for her.

And now with the diabetes, she tells everyone, "I just a diabetes girl" and shrugs her shoulders and smiles. She tries to explain to people about it—how they have to test her blood sugars and she gets insulin and has to watch what she eats, etc. She does often say, "I not know why I got diabetes?" but it's as much rhetorical as anything. She shed some tears and certainly has needed extra hugs this past week but really has been remarkable. She gets mad about having to have insulin and tried to bargain her way out of it the first few days but hasn't the past couple of days; in fact, she comes up and asks if it is time for blood sugar or insulin or one of her meals. We've tried to give her as much self-determination as we can (such as letting her pick which finger to prick, who gives her the shot, etc.) and that seems to help.

Whitney is very aware of her differences though and very conscious of how other people treat her. But I think that time has proven to her that the people that aren't accepting of her (and other children or individuals like her) are the ones who are the losers, not her.

She will get frustrated at times if she can't do things like ride a bike but we've always tried to remind her that there are other people without any other challenges who can't ride bikes or whatever it is she may be focusing on. And that's always satisfied her. She may talk about it for awhile and try to sort the pieces out but then she just seems to do just that and moves on.

She does talk about what she wants to be when she grows up and all that—we try not to put limitations on her future because there's still so much to be determined but it's interesting that she talks about things like her and I having a day care or working in a store or things like that. She positively insists that she does not want to go to college. So it's almost as though she has some cognitive sense of the future given her situation.

She never really has gotten too mad about not being able to do something—certainly frustrated at times but she has this incredible sense of inner motivation or self-confidence or serenity (who knows what it is) that takes over and focuses more on the positives than the negatives. (I feel like this is sounding terribly Pollyanna-ish but it's really always been the case.) We talk about feelings a lot and try to help her articulate any frustration, anger, and how it's absolutely okay to feel that way. That's its okay to stomp her feet or feel "steamin' mad" as she says but that you have to deal with it in acceptable ways—like not slamming doors (We're not 100 percent successful of course!)

Lauren

Following an uncomplicated pregnancy, our beautiful daughter Lauren was delivered into the world on May 2, 1994. She weighed 7 pounds, 3 ounces and was 20 inches long. There were no immediate neonatal problems, and Lauren went home at 2 days of age. As new parents, we felt a lot of joy and excitement, and a little bit of anxiety. She was so small and innocent and was completely dependent on us.

Lauren's first two months of life consisted of eating and sleeping and being watched over by two loving and proud parents. It wasn't until her 2 month check up that there appeared to be a problem with Lauren's vision. Lauren's pediatrician noticed that her eyes jumped around in a chaotic fashion, and she did not follow or focus on objects. She was immediately scheduled to see a pediatric opthamologist.

During Lauren's visit with the opthamologist, her eyes were dilated for better viewing of the optic nerve. The doctor wanted to verify the connections of the optic nerve to rule out any concerns in this area. No conclusions were made from this visit, although Lauren was diagnosed with Hyperopia, Exotropia and Congenital Nystagmus.

Lauren was then scheduled for a CAT Scan for an even better view of the optic nerve, and to rule out the possibility of a brain tumor. The CAT Scan was unremarkable, and again no conclusive diagnosis was made. As parents, we felt a small degree of relief, but were still very concerned about what was going on with our little daughter and her vision.

An MRI was scheduled for Lauren the next day, and

an appointment with a pediatric neurologist was to follow. The MRI demonstrated hypoplasia of the cerebellar vermis. Along with Lauren's visual limitations and cerebellar vermis abnormality, the neurologist gave Lauren the diagnosis of Joubert Syndrome.

Lauren was also scheduled for special eye tests—a Visual Evoked Response (VER) and an Electroretinography (ERG). The results of these tests were very discouraging: we were told that Lauren may never have vision.

Because there is not a great deal of information available about Joubert Syndrome, and many physicians have never heard of the disorder, we were left with many questions about Lauren's future. We also had very strong feelings of guilt. What did we do or not do during the pregnancy that would have helped her to avoid this condition.

Shortly after the diagnosis was made, we met with a Geneticist. At that appointment we learned a little bit about Joubert Syndrome, but the information that was available was both limited and discouraging. At the visit, we all gave blood which was sent to a research lab in Philadelphia, Pennsylvania. After meeting with the pediatric geneticist, we learned that we could not have done anything differently to prevent Joubert Syndrome. Lauren wore eye glasses for about a year to correct her farsightedness. At each visit with the eye doctor, the degree of farsightedness decreased to the point where Lauren no longer needed to wear glasses. Despite the earlier progosis, and the VER and ERG test results, Lauren's visual abilities have improved significantly.

After learning of Lauren's diagnosis, we immediately checked into what services were available for Lauren to help her develop physically as well as intellectually. We contacted Early Intervention and began a therapy program for Lauren. She originally received Physical Therapy and Occupational Therapy 2 days each week. This was increased to 4 days each week with the inclusion of Speech Therapy. Separate therapy was also coordinated for Lauren through our health insurance plan. As a convenience to us, and to promote a better environment for Lauren, all services were provided to Lauren in the day care she was enrolled in. This allowed the therapists to educate us as well as the day care staff on various techniques they could use with Lauren to continue her therapy at other times throughout the day.

Lauren also attended a Feeding Clinic on one occasion. At that time she was not chewing solid foods. Part of her difficulties with eating were a result of her constant tongue protrusion (which she no longer does). During the session, we primarily learned more appropriate ways to feed her to encourage her to take a more active role in the processing of food. This made a tremendous difference in her eating abilities.

At the recommendation of Lauren's Physical Therapist, we ordered and received a Tumbleform Tristander. We used this piece of equipment with Lauren as much as possible. She has since outgrown the need to use this equipment; however, it made a significant difference in Lauren's tolerance of weight bearing.

When Lauren turned 3 years old, she was no longer eligible to receive Early Intervention services. After much research and several site visits, Lauren was enrolled in a program funded by the school district. She attends a special needs program from 9:00 a.m. to 3:00 p.m. Through the school program, Lauren receives many therapies on a daily basis, and we continue to take Lauren to focused PT, OT and ST sessions several times each week (through our health insurance plan). Lauren has progressed in ways we could have only hoped for several years ago.

Lauren communicates primarily through few words which only we understand, and the use of sign language. Lauren knows at least 150 words and uses it to communicate her wants and needs. Lauren is also beginning to use an Augmentative Communication Device both at school and at home (which was paid for by the school district) to vocalize her wants. Our goal with the "talker" is that she will be encouraged to try to make more sounds and form more words with her own voice.

Lauren is a smart, happy, beautiful 4½ year old who is now crawling, sitting up, playing and eating independently. She loves to read books, watch Barney and play with her baby sister Ashley. We are confident that she will walk and talk some day soon as she is determined to do all the things "unaffected" children do, and she has a strong will to succeed. We still have concerns about her future and often experience pangs of guilt about if we are doing what is best for Lauren, but we would never change the past. We have learned to accept our blessings and no longer take the small things in life for granted.

We first learned about the Parents In Touch Network by pure luck. My Aunt was a Medical Technologist in a Hospital in Pittsburgh, PA. When we learned of the diagnosis, my mother called her sister to see if she knew of Joubert Syndrome. She did not, but she asked around at the hospital. No one knew anything about it, including the doctors. One of the nurses she spoke with told my Aunt that she had a patient in the hospital who had a son with Joubert Syndrome. She told her that her son was diagnosed and was given a bleak prognosis; however, he proved the doctors wrong. His mother was told he would never see, walk, talk, etc., and he was doing all those things. My Aunt was then given the name of Mary Van Damme to contact to learn more about the Network.

Lauren's most difficult obstacle to date has been her balance. She wants to walk, but can not steady herself in the prone position. This has been difficult for us as well because as Lauren grows up and gets heavier, she is more difficult to carry around (although we do use her wheelchair whenever we can).

Our biggest concern about Lauren's education is whether she is challenged enough in the school she attends. Lauren attends a Cerebral Palsy center which has many children (and adults) with various disabilities (not just CP) and varying degrees of needs. Lauren also attends a day care program before and after school which integrates her with regular children. We are waiting to see how the rest of the school year is, and when Lauren turns 5 in May, we are considering evaluating regular kindergarten classes to see if Lauren may benefit more being integrated into a regular school program.

Abby

I had a normal pregnancy for the most part. I did experience an unusual sensation. It was a strong flutter or spasm in my belly that I knew wasn't coming from my body. It occurred about 5 or 6 times, the first one being in my 5th month of pregnancy. I had been pregnant before and was pretty sure this wasn't normal. But, I did not want to believe anything was wrong, so I ignored it. When Abby was born she was not breathing and was completely limp. She had to be resuscitated. When Abby started breathing, she did so at a very rapid rate, which I'd never seen before in any child. I knew right away that her breathing pattern was the reason I felt those spasms. The doctors and nurses weren't sure why she was breathing so fast, but told us that sometimes preemies will breathe fast for a few hours. They tried to reassure us that she would be fine, but her breathing never normalized.

Abby was a big baby, weighing in at 9lbs 7oz and 22 inches long. The day after she was born she was transferred to another hospital that had a Neonatal Intensive Care Unit. She looked huge compared to all the preemies in the NICU. For the next seven days she had more tests done than most people do in a lifetime. One of her tests was an MRI and a doctor took this test with him to the University Hospital (he had rotations at three hospitals) and showed it to a pediatric neurologist. The neurologist made a tentative diagnosis of Joubert Syndrome and set us up for an appointment in his office six weeks later. Because doctors in the NICU didn't know what else to do for Abby, they sent her home. Abby had apnea along with her hyperpnea every twenty seconds or so. She never stopped breathing long enough to turn blue, but the hospital sent an apnea monitor home with her. We were fortunate that she had good suck and swallow reflexes, although she would choke on her milk two or three times every time she nursed. (It took a few months for her to coordinate her rapid breathing with swallowing.)

At home, the apnea monitor's alarm went off every few minutes, because it just couldn't recognize Abby's breathing pattern. We were exhausted from loss of sleep due to the monitor going off and from the stress of having something seriously wrong with our precious baby. We decided jointly to give the monitor back after a week. She hadn't turned blue at any time in her first two weeks of life and we just hoped and prayed that she wouldn't after the monitor was gone. We had to get some sleep. Well, that was the plan anyway. Abby slept no longer than two hours at any one time. (This continued for months.) Her apnea disturbed her sleep and she kept waking up and crying. The only way she would fall back to sleep was by rocking her.

When Abby was about three weeks old, she started crying for two to three hours at a time, about every other day. (We didn't realize at first that this was the beginning of a colicky period that would last until she was four and a half months old.) Within a week she was crying for six hours at a time. She would usually start crying around 11:00 pm and cry for two hours, nurse for ten minutes, sleep for ten minutes, then wake up and start that all over again. Most of her crying episodes were about six hours long, with her worst bout lasting twelve hours. When Abby was four weeks old, we took her to the University Hospital for another MRI. (The neurologist who had made the tentative diagnosis of JS wasn't sure if Abby had part of her vermis, so he wanted to get another picture of her brain. The second test was also inconclusive.) That night, after we had returned home, she cried for hours and had trouble catching her breath. We took her to back to the University Hospital, this time to the emergency room. Although she had fallen asleep from exhaustion and was breathing better by the time doctors examined her, she was admitted to the hospital. One doctor did a sleep study on her because of her apnea and learned that her oxygen level dipped during each apneatic period. He prescribed ½ liter of continuous oxygen. While Abby was there, the neurologist made the diagnosis of Joubert Syndrome. Five months earlier this neurologist had diagnosed another baby with JS. This was fortunate for us because it may have taken much longer to get the correct diagnosis. Of course no one could tell us much past the fact that it was called Joubert Syndrome. (One geneticist did tell me that she was retarded. I still don't understand how he could have known that when she was only four weeks old and he had never heard of Joubert Syndrome until Abby came along.) This time Abby was sent home from the hospital with oxygen. This wasn't as annoying as the apnea monitor.

We were stunned with the diagnosis. Even though we knew in our heads that something was wrong with Abby, we hoped in our hearts that her problem would go away with time. Now her problem had a name and it was time to move on to the next step.

At the suggestion of the neurologist, we called the early intervention program (Early On) run by our school system. We signed her up when she was four months old. A therapist and special education teacher came to our house once a week to work with her and show me how I could help her. Although I hated the idea of needing them, I was still grateful to have their help. Abby's progress was very slow. Since I already had a child three years older than Abby, I knew Abby was missing many milestones. She rolled over for the first time at ten months, and it was still exciting, even though it was so late. (Now, at age three, she rolls around easily, but will not yet attempt to crawl. We are still working on sitting, also.)

Her breathing and apnea pattern improved a little at around 14 months. She was able to sleep longer periods of time at night, although her daytime naps were usually only 45 minutes long. (But she didn't sleep through the night until about age two and a half.)

I started recognizing a pattern in Abby around her first birthday. She had "good cycles" and "bad cycles". Her bad cycles would usually last four to six weeks, where she had tachypnea more often and would be irritable and uncooperative with therapy. She wanted to be rocked by her mother all the time. It was so comforting to her (but tiring to mom). Then, she would go into a good cycle, lasting three or four weeks, where she was happier, more willing to do therapy and had less tachypnea. (That pattern isn't so prevalent now at age three, but she still has "cycles" that are less predictable.)

She is eligible for preschool this fall, and we are fortunate that there is a great school nearby for severely handicapped children. Although we feel she is smart enough to go to other "special needs" preschools, the one she will be attending will give her the therapy she needs, since she is so far behind in physical development. She also has no speech, has feeding problems and can barely sit. We just started working on sign language. She can sign "more" and we are working on other words, too. Her preschool will be helping her with signing, also. We hope to see more progress with Abby this year, since she will be getting therapy away from home as well.

Although the road has been a bumpy one, we have learned a lot about life from Abby. We have become more patient and understanding, more accepting of other people and less tolerant to prejudice. If life's road was easy, we wouldn't grow as much.

Will

Dear Family and Friends:

As many of you know we've had one big eventful year. I want to tell you about what has been happening in our lives so that you will understand and will not be afraid to ask us questions. I am not sure where or how to begin telling all that we have learned this year; however, first of all, we want you to know how much we appreciate your support, thoughtful notes, gifts, phone calls, encouraging words, visits, and prayers.

After many years of hoping for children and several more years of fertility testing and surgeries and a miscarriage, we had given up our hope of becoming parents when I found out I was seven weeks pregnant. If all went well we would be parents at the end of April 1995. We were thrilled. I had a very easy pregnancy until the seventh month when a Level II ultrasound indicated an area of underdevelopment in the third and fourth ventricles of our baby's brain. After speaking with a genetic counselor we immediately made an appointment with a neurologist to find out what the implications could be. The physician told us that the finding might not mean anything or could mean that our baby would need a shunt for hydrocephalus. He let us know that we could not know the severity of the condition until the little guy was born. He recommended that we make an appointment with a pediatrician who treats children with similar conditions.

We made the appointment for 5:30 p.m. on April 10, 1995. On April 9, at 2:00 p.m. my water broke. We were in labor for more than ten hours when the OBGYN decided to do a C-section. Our baby Will was born at 11:53 p.m. weighing 7lbs. 13.4 oz. and was 21.5 inches long. We heard a very tiny squeak when they laid him on the warmer (a tray with a heater, blankets, and lights used to keep neonates warm). He was having trouble breathing and was intubated immediately. Wayne got the first look at him, but I was not able to see him until the next morning when they were transporting him to a neonatal intensive care unit at another local hospital. I fell in love with him at first sight. He looked like his daddy. He had red hair and the same shape to his hands as Wayne's.

It was awful not being able to hold him, but I knew he needed the expertise of the doctors to help him get stronger. We were scared. I was dismissed from the hospital on April 11, and made a straight line for the NICU where they were holding my baby. Will was taking about 110 breaths per minute (bpm) when I first saw him. The normal range for bpm is 20 to 60. We held him for as long as we were allowed to visit. It broke our hearts to leave him each night. We cried buckets and buckets of tears. We cried over the irrational thoughts that Will's condition had something to do with something we ate, didn't eat, were exposed to, or could have prevented. We felt so inadequate to be parents. We got mad at our ignorance of the medical field. We decided that since we both hurt so much that we could not be mad at each other.

After four weeks in the hospital and many training sessions in feeding Will through a nasal-gastric/oral gastric (NG/OG) tube, and a bottle, we were allowed to bring him home. As we were gathering our supplies and things for home, a doctor came to us and told us that she thought that Will had severe reflux and that he may aspirate. To aspirate means that food or stomach content is inhaled into the lungs usually resulting in death. We had the choice to take him on home with the risk of aspiration, or to send him in for surgery to have a fundalplication and the placement of a Gastrostomy tube (G-tube). Since he had not aspirated in the four and one half weeks he spent in the NICU, and since he was sucking from a bottle, gaining weight, and we were able to place the NG/OG tubes ourselves, we decided to take him on home. We were given an apnea and heart monitor and several prescriptions for the reflux and breathing problems.

Our days filled with round the clock three hour feedings. After the third week home, Will's monitor started beeping a low heart rate signal. I noticed that he was not breathing. Wayne laid him on the floor and began CPR while I called 911. Will came around before the ambulance arrived. The EMT, assured us that we had done the right thing, examined Will and thought that he would be okay at home. The EMT reviewed CPR with us, called our pediatrician for us and then called every two or three hours throughout the day to check on Will. Will seemed okay.

Then, on the fifth week that we had him home, the neurologist thought that we should see a geneticist who thought she knew what was happening with Will. She told us that she suspected that Will had Joubert Syndrome and would never walk or talk and would surely die before age two. She also told us that she did not know much about the syndrome but one of her colleagues had done extensive work in the subject and would be able to talk to us in four weeks. We were devastated. We could barely take our own breath realizing that our baby could die at any moment. Thank goodness for our pediatrician, Dr. C, who noticed some of the good things about Will that were inconsistent with a fatal diagnosis. He encouraged us to keep gathering information and to rule out the diagnosis.

Three more weeks passed. One week we spent another four days in the pediatric intensive care unit because Will again quit breathing. I was by myself and somehow gave him CPR and called 911. This time we were told that he had RSV which is a respiratory infection similar to pneumonia type infections. We were released after four days.

The following week we met with the geneticist who had done the research with Joubert Syndrome. He agreed with the diagnosis but told us there was hope for Will's life. He explained that there is a wide spectrum of severity in persons with Joubert Syndrome. Besides the reality of many children with the syndrome who die of respiratory complications, he knew of two cases of thirty year old males who could walk, talk, and one of them had completed college and a master's degree. Furthermore, he told us that by working with speech, physical, and occupational therapists, and by using monitors for the apnea, we could expect a better chance for Will's life. In addition, he gave us a brief description of the genetic disorder explaining that Joubert Syndrome is an autosomal recessive trait in which both parents have to be recessive gene carriers to have a child with Joubert Syndrome. He convincingly assured us that Will's condition was not due to anything we had eaten, done (such as getting older), or the result of any kind of chemical to which we had been exposed. He further stated that our baby's condition is a genetic factor of which we have no control.

Feeling more hopeful about our little boy, another three weeks passed filled with visits from family members who tried to help us with the three hour feeding schedule and the constant holding Will required to help him with his reflux and apnea problems. Friends sent food to us. We could not have survived without their help. Not only were we grieving the loss of our dream of a "perfect child", we were giving all we had to keep up with his prescribed schedule, the "new baby" responsibilities, and his special medical needs.

Again on July 5th, Will stopped breathing. Fortunately, my sister was visiting and called Dr. C while I gave Will puffs of breath and a few chest compressions. Wayne rushed home from work and drove us to Dr. C's office. Dr. C decided that he would like for us to see the specialists at Children's Medical Center (CMC) in Atlanta. Will and I took the four hour ambulance ride while Wayne followed behind in the car. Actually, Wayne got ahead of the ambulance and was already there when we arrived. Will was put on a respirator that night and was again diagnosed with RSV.

During our ten week stay at CMC, Will had a physician assigned to every one of his body systems. We met all kinds of "-ologists". After many medical tests, severe reflux and the absolute risk of aspiration were validated. The fundalplication was done and a Gastrostomy tube was placed in Will's abdomen. A fundalplication is a surgical procedure in which the upper part of the stomach, the fundus, is wrapped around the lower part of esophagus to keep stomach content from being regurgitated or refluxed. The G-tube enables us to feed Will without him having to work so hard at coordinating his swallow and possibly aspirating. Note, it is important not to confuse a G-tube with a G-string. That is something else for another part of the anatomy. The surgeon who placed the Gastrostomy tube was a bit disturbed when he overheard me tell a nurse that he had fitted Will with a G-string. There is quite a difference in the connotation of the terms. Nonetheless, we think that the G-tube will allow Will the energy for growth and development rather than using all his energy in getting enough food.

Although being in the intensive care units at CMC was not how we had planned to spend our Summer 1995, our stay there gave us the opportunity to research and correspond with the Joubert Syndrome Parents-In-Touch Network. Thus, according to research, one in 250 people are carriers. There is a 25% chance of two carriers having an affected child. My brothers and sisters and Wayne's sister have a 50% chance of being carriers; however, their mates have a 1 in 250% chance. The possibility of them having an affected child is 1 in 2,000. Approximately, 1 in 200,000 children are born with Joubert Syndrome. At the time of his diagnosis, May 1995, Will was the fourth child in the state of Georgia known to have Joubert's.

In other reports we have found that Joubert Syndrome is a rare genetic disorder in which there are congenital problems which fit into a recognizable pattern of features. The most typical characteristic of the syndrome is the absence or underdevelopment of part of the brain called the cerebellar vermis that causes a problem with coordination and balance. Another characteristic is a malformed brainstem which causes an abnormal breathing pattern called episodic hypernea, in which babies pant, and may be followed by apnea (the cessation of breathing), abnormal eye and tongue movements, and hypotonia (low tone in the muscles). All of these characteristics contribute to delays in development. Other physical malformations that may occur involve extra fingers and toes, cleft lip or palate, tongue abnormalities, and seizures.

The prognosis for Joubert Syndrome is developmental delays such as sitting, head control, crawling, walking, and talking; however, health and growth are not usually affected. Commonly there is a degree of mild or moderate retardation. Again the severity has a wide spectrum. There are a few cases of affected individuals with normal intelligence or learning disabilities. The geneticist we spoke with in June explained that since writing and talking are the most used methods to determine intelligence, and since these children have difficulty coordinating their muscles for writing and speaking, they often score low on IQ tests. However, with new technology and a variety of different ways of communication, more recent studies indicate that many of these children are of normal intelligence.

In relation to the research, an MRI and CAT SCAN taken of Will indicate cerebellar vermis hypoplasia or underdevelopment of the vermis. Although he presently breaths at a much more even rate (approximately 20-40bpm) during the first six months be exhibited episodic hypernea, tachypnea (irregular breathing pattern), and prolonged apnoeic attacks often lasting over thirty seconds. He still has what several physicians describe as breath holding spells which require resuscitative breathing and sometimes several rounds of CPR. These breath holding episodes which we call "clamp downs" usually occur when Will is in pain from a plugged nostril, teething, stomach, or gas in his intestinal track. He does not have extra digits, and as far as our entourage of physicians can tell, he does not have the kidney or liver complications. He is hypotonic. This low body tone seems to have an effect on muscles that I never even thought about such as those of the throat, tongue, digestive tract, face, and eyes. He barely opened his eyelids the first month of his life. It was not until he was three months old that he began to keep his eyes open. He does not track with his eyes and appears to focus only occasionally. An ERG (electroretinogram) showed that he does have some connections between his retina and the vision center of his brain; however there were some areas, or planes of vision which showed very low or no vision. A second ERG indicated outer ring retinal dystrophy. We are unsure of how much Will can see, but know that he does not see very much because of the retina complication. Other test indicate normal hearing. He quiets to music, voices, and the purr of our eight year old cat, Rudy. Will turns his head in the direction of sound, kicks his legs to the beat of the music, and makes popping sounds with his lips, hums, and says ma-ma-ma, de-de, na-na, ren-ren, and no. When he was seven months old, Wayne and I were sitting in Will's room listening to his baby babbling and distinctly heard Will say, "na-na dooo-ing". We laughed because we know that we have constantly asked him, "what are you doing?", whenever his monitors alarm.

The periods of sound-making seem to come and go with Will. Lately, he has not made many sounds other than grunts and squeals. He has been teething and since he cannot hold onto something to bite; he bites the nearest thing to his gums—his tongue. This has caused him some pain, and has caused us a tremendous amount of worry. We were able to find a dentist who ground off the sharp edges to Will's five teeth. That helped tremendously, but every other day his tongue gets caught in between his "mighty jaws", and we have another injury. We are stumped with what to do about the problem but have discovered a few possible solutions. Over these past few weeks, he has been less interested in biting on his tongue and has given us clearer signals to indicate that it is "biting time".

Presently, we are part of a research project to find the gene that causes Joubert Syndrome. Finding the gene will most likely not help Will's condition but may help others who could benefit from gene therapy. In June 1996, we left Will in the care of his nurses, my aunt, and Wayne's mom while we traveled to Chicago and attended a conference for parents of children with the syndrome. At the conference we met many of the leading physicians, researchers and therapists who are working to find answers and solutions for the problems associated with the syndrome. We even met the geneticist, Dr. Marie Joubert, who first described the syndrome at a Canadian hospital in 1969. The conference allowed us the opportunity to meet other parents and learn from their experiences. Since Will's birth, we have seen thirty physicians and several of those have been specialists. In April 1996, we visited two physicians in Gainesville, Florida who have been researching children and families with Joubert Syndrome. We learned from them that the syndrome is not a digressive disease. Children with JS tend to get stronger; however, we must be "cautiously optimistic". Another physician told us that usually 80% of babies with JS die before their first birthday, and of the 20% left, 50% of them die within the second year; but, of the children who survive through the second year there is greater chance of a normal life span.

At sixteen months, Will can sit supported, sat unsupported for three whole seconds last week, can roll from side to side, and from back to tummy, and tummy to back (when he wants to, or when he can). He smiles, chuckles, and laughs. He plays "hide and seek" by rolling to his side, closing his eyes (so we can't see him), and then waits for someone to say "where is Will?" before he rolls to his back, kicks his legs, and grins at us. He held a rattle and moved it all by himself several times during this past month. He has not shown signs of being tactile or orally defensive. He does not take food by mouth but enjoys biting on a bite block we designed using a spongy boat key float and waterproof tape. He likes to be held, rocked, and talked to. He seems to enjoy music and will "dance" by kicking either reciprocally with both legs, or by moving just one leg to the beat of the music. Good songs get both legs going up and down, the others are just "one-legged" songs. We have worked with a physical therapist and will soon begin working with both occupational and speech therapists. We have used a local organization's vision therapist to stimulate Will's vision capacity and to gain the knowledge needed for teaching a baby who has low vision.

We don't know where our chances for Will's life fall on the percentage tables and charts shown in the literature about Joubert Syndrome. We do know that we are thankful for every day that we can be together. We also know that there have been many blessings to count and special persons that we have met because of our experience. We do not feel persecuted by God or fate. We feel blessed. Along with many other parents of children with disabilities, we feel that we would not have chosen this to be, but can not imagine that our lives would be any richer had we not begun our travel down the road with a child of special needs. We do what we have to do, and we take each day one by one, and often, minute by minute. We believe in the scripture Romans 8:28.

Update: At the time of printing, Will was waiting to celebrate his sixth birthday. He was also on a kidney transplant list.

Joey

It all began on the day Michael and I were married: November 8, 1992. We both wanted children right away and that is exactly what we got. By February 1993, I was pregnant and was expecting around the time of our first wedding anniversary.

When we learned that we were going to be parents, we were excited but scared at the same time thinking that this child would depend on us for everything. Then we would question ourselves "Would we be good parents to this child?" and "Would we raise him/her to be a good person in this world?" I guess these are common questions first time parents ask themselves but for us, it was all new.

The doctors' appointments were definitely exciting. Going in every month, hearing things about the baby, hearing the heartbeat, and seeing pictures up on the wall of the stage our child was at. We took all the normal routine tests that go along in pregnancy. The routine urine test when you go in, eventually the Triple-Marker, the famous diabetic test where you drink that really sweet syrup and then they test your sugar level and then between 18–20 weeks the first ultra sound. We were very excited about the ultrasound. There was something about getting to see what our baby looked like so early in the game. Mike's mom and my mother, along with Mike and I were at the ultrasound. After drinking all that water and then the technician pushing on my stomach you would think that I would have released my bladder right then and there, but seeing the first glimpse of our little baby made all that go away. He was as precious as could be. Everything looked normal from head to toe. The baby even woke up a little bit and moved for us. We got pictures and a little bit of video. We bought it home and would look at the pictures and the video and were amazed that this human life was living and growing inside of me.

The remainder of the pregnancy was normal. At week 34, my doctor wanted to do another routine ultrasound. Everything looked fine but she was a little concerned that the placenta was maturing too fast and that the baby was not getting enough nutrition. She did say that there was enough amniotic fluid there and not to be too concerned but to come back in a week to check and see what was going on.

We went back the next week, and she asked the normal questions, "Is the baby still active?" "Have the movements changed in anyway?" Again I said, "No, everything has been the same." We proceeded to do the ultra sound. The technician always checked the baby from head to toe even if they were looking for just one thing. This time when he looked at the head he noticed something dark. He called the doctor in and she was a bit concerned and said that it was probably nothing but would like me to see a specialist that would do a Level II ultrasound to give us a clearer picture.

We made the appointment and went to Santa Monica. She did an abdominal view and said everything looks great. Sometimes there are shadows that appear that are really not problems. She would have to do a vaginal ultrasound since she could not see the other side of the head. At this point we were thinking we were in the clear. She began looking and said, "Yes I see something." Now my heart was racing and I wanted to know more. She said that there was a cyst on the 4th ventricle; an enlarged 4th ventricle and encephaloseal (where the skull did not fuse together and the meninges [thin membranes that cover the brain] were exposed). At this point we were in shock. She gave the diagnosis of Dandy Walker Syndrome and proceeded to tell us that he would need a shunt placed in the ventricle where tubing would be placed and go down into the stomach in order for the cerebral spinal fluid (CSF) to drain properly. She also said that they would place a few stitches in the occipital region (lower portion of the back of the head) after birth and then the skull would fuse together. At this point and time we were so devastated that we wanted to hear something good so we asked if she could tell what the gender was. She said that we were having a boy.

She then explained that this child should not be born vaginally. He should be delivered cesarean section (c-section) as they did not want any pressure on the baby's head. She requested an amniocentesis to see if the baby's lungs were ready for delivery. Still being in shock of hearing everything, I kept wondering if this was a terrible dream and wanted to wake up so badly. While driving home I told Mike that if he wanted to divorce me and get remarried and have normal kids with someone else I would understand. He immediately pulled the car over and said "NO! We are in this together and I love you and my son no matter what. Do not ever say that again!" And I never have.

We went back to our doctor where she had hospital rights and did the amnio. The preliminary results would be given early in the evening and the final results would be later that night. They scheduled a c-section for the next morning, which was a Friday just in case his lungs were ready. Meanwhile, my baby shower was that Saturday afternoon. I was worried what to say to people at the shower. Mike said not to worry, that things would work out and that right now, the baby and I were more important. Approximately 11:00pm that Thursday night, my OBGYN called and said that the baby's lungs were not ready and they would monitor the situation and wait until the baby was 38 ½ weeks before he was delivered. They did not want to deliver a child with neurological problems and respiratory problems as well.

The baby shower went as planned. We did not tell anyone that we knew there were problems other than our close families. As I sat there opening up presents, I felt as if I were miles away. I could hear everyone's voices around me as if I were off in the distance even though they were sitting right next to me. Later, after Joey was born, my best friend said that she had noticed that something was wrong with me that day but didn't know what.

I was monitored for stress as well as the baby. Everything was going along well. We were right in the middle of getting our new house ready for us to move into before the baby was born but during those next three weeks all I could do was think that maybe none of this was true. That I should just wait and see what happens the day the baby is born. Since we knew the delivery was going to be a c-section, we got to pick the date. We decided on November 22, 1993. It had a nice ring to it and it also happened to be the 25th anniversary of John F. Kennedy's death.

Before we knew it, the day had arrived. I still remember waking up that morning and not wanting to go through with the delivery. I couldn't help but feel that he was safe where he was now and he could just stay inside me. We arrived at the hospital at 5:30 am. I was hooked up to monitors and IV's were stuck in me and then prepped for surgery. I walked to the c-section operating room in one of their sexy hospital gowns that tie in the back with my backside in plain view. I walked by the nurses' station and there also happens to be all the doctors that were going to be involved in this c-section. Our pediatrician (which happened to be my pediatrician when I was a child) insisted on being there for the delivery, an ultrasound technician was there to do scans of the baby's head after birth, and of course, the wonderful anesthesiologist who not only gives you the epidural but that wonderful drug morphine and many many more that I cannot remember. It seemed like there were tons of people in there and Mike was the only family that I could have with me.

With everything in place, the surgery began and Joseph was born at 7:44 am. I could hear him crying and the doctors said he looked good. He weighted 7lbs 9ozs and was 20 ½ inches long. After Mike cut the cord, they bundled him up with a cap on and Mike sat there holding him next to me. After looking at him I realized that the ultra sound technician had been wrong. There were no meninges out like she said and so I thought that everything was prefect. Mike went with Joey to the Nursery and I was being sewed up. The only thing I remember after that was saying that I was not feeling too good and can I have the oxygen mask back. I woke up in the recovery room with Mike beside me. I was freezing and wanted more blankets. They said this was a normal side effect.

Later that day, I learned that forty-five minutes after Joey was born while in the nursery he stopped breathing and turned blue. He was rushed over to NICU. They used an ambu bag on him to get him breathing again. He was placed in an oxygen hood and then hooked up to monitors. I was not allowed to get up out of bed since I had just had surgery. Mike would go and see him and report back to me. The nurses took Polaroid's and sent them to me so I could see him. That night I asked Mike to spend the night there since they had given me a private suite. I know they knew it would not be good to place me in a regular room along with another mother that had a healthy child. So Mike slept on the sofa bed. In the middle of the night I heard CODE BLUE..... CODE BLUE!!! I sat up and started yelling to Mike to go and check on Joey. I knew something had happened. Mike ran down there and he was doing just fine. He asked the nurse why a code blue would be announced like that and she told him that it should not have been announced on our floor. Talk about a heart attack!

The next day I was up walking a little bit and was able to get in a wheelchair to go see our beautiful Joey. It was also time to feed him. They told me that he was having problems feeding. He would suck and swallow and not breathe. You had to take the bottle out and let him take a breath and then begin to feed him again. He also had some tissue growths on his tongue and they thought that maybe that contributed to the eating problem. This was the first time I got to hold our little Joey. He was very precious. I gave him a bottle and boy did he suck and swallow but he did not stop to take a breath. You would pull it out and he would begin to breath and then you would place the bottle back and he would suck and swallow away. At some point they placed a Nasogastric Tube (n-tube, a tube placed down through the nose into the stomach) They also said they saw some seizure activity, a quivering chin, on Joey and placed him on an anticonvulsant. They did an EEG and that came back normal. They also said they heard something weird with his heart and that maybe he had a hole in his heart. They did an EKG and that came back normal as well. So, all these tests and everything so far was coming back normal.

Day Three, he went in for an MRI. When we got the results, we were told that there were some pieces missing, the ventricle was enlarged and there was a cyst. The Neonatologist also told us that Joey would never do anything but lie there. She sent in some people from an institution to talk to us about placing Joey there. I spoke up and said, “Wait! This child is only three days old and you are giving up on him already? He deserves a chance.” She had basically written him off. We had met her once before, during the amnio, and her bedside manners then were not good either.

Day Four was Thanksgiving and I was released from the hospital. It was very hard for me to leave our little Joey there. I was wheeled out in a wheelchair like other mothers are when they are leaving the hospital except I was carrying a blue fluffy teddy bear that was brought to the hospital for Joey.

By that Friday, at five days old, there was nothing more they could do at this hospital and wanted to transfer him to Children's in Los Angeles. We had an appointment with a Neurosurgeon that Monday. We spent all of Friday, Saturday and Sunday at the hospital. We did come home and sleep but would return early in the morning. He was pretty stable. He did breathe fast at times and the feeding was still an issue. He also would have apnea spells and therefore was placed on oxygen. We heard from the Neurosurgeon and he said that there would be no need for a shunt since the cerebrospinal fluid was draining properly and the ventricle in question was simply enlarged. We never did meet him face to face.

Much of this was and still is a blur. I remember going and sitting in a rocking chair for hours holding Joey and rocking him. There were times we would walk up to the window at the nursery and see that Joey was NOT lying there and panic. Since Joey was the only child not hooked up to tons of equipment, nurses would take him out, hold him and walk around with him. I was also told that a volunteer, an older lady, would come and sit and rock Joey late at night when we were not there. I never got to meet that woman but they said she took a liking to Joey. We need more people in the world like that.

I believe it was during the second week of Joey's stay that a Geneticist came in to see Joey and said he believed that Joey had Joubert Syndrome but he would like to run a few more tests. After hearing this, we talked to our pediatrician. He looked up Joubert Syndrome and when he read what was written we all said that Joey did not have JS based on the characteristics in the readings. We also had a conference with a dozen doctors. We sat down with them in a meeting room and the head Neurologist said, "Tell us what it is you think is going on with your son." Mike proceeded to tell them everything that we knew and I would fill in where he would forget information. After a twenty-minute talk from Mike and me, the head doctor said "I do not know why we had this meeting. You know what we know about your son. You are two intelligent people and Joey is very lucky to have you both. We still have the feeding issue that will be addressed by the surgeon right now." The nurse presented what she had and then the surgeon suggested that a gastrostomy tube (g-tube) be placed in for eating. They said that it was a wise decision since they did not want him going home with the N-tube.

We met with the surgeon and signed all the necessary paper work for the surgery. They also coordinated with an Ear, Nose and Throat (ENT) doctor to be in this procedure so he could laser off the growths and also do a scope down his throat to see if there were any growths down his throat. The surgery went well with the G-tube and the laser surgery went well too. The ENT did report that there were no growths down the throat but he did find that Joey had paralyzed vocal chords. We said "Why can we hear him when he cries?" He replied, "The reason is because they are paralyzed in the closed position and that is what causes the sound, the vibration of the chords." He also stated that usually chords are paralyzed in the open position. He said he did not know if his chords would work again. He was not sure of the cause of the paralysis. It could have been because of the neurological problems or it could have been from the birth. We informed him that Joey was delivered very carefully and that we thought that there was no damage done at birth. He said he was not sure if they would come back or not but to wait for the one month check up. He did comment that since the chords were in the closed position that is why there were times that Joey was having a hard time breathing and was noisy. He had wanted to do a tracheotomy and we said no. We mentioned to him that Joey does reposition his head to breathe better and when the doctor saw that, he decided to hold off until the next check-up.

Four days after the surgery on December 10,1993, Joey finally came home with us. We had oxygen and an apnea monitor along with us. We were both very nervous bringing home this little baby with this equipment. We knew how to feed Joey since the nurses at the hospital would show us what to do and then let us feed him. They told us we could call them anytime if we had questions which we did at first but as the weeks went on the calls were less and less.

January 17, 1994 was a scary moment for us. Joey had only been home about 5 weeks when at 4:31 am PST the Northridge earthquake hit. We had just finished feeding Joey at 4:25 am and we laid him between us in our bed. All of a sudden, we were awoken by a huge jolt. It felt like someone picked up our house and was standing there shaking it up and down. I covered up Joey and Mike covered me and he had a pillow over his head. After the shaking quit, which seemed like forever, and after trying to find a flashlight, we saw that my dresser had fallen over and a drawer was lying right where Joey would have been if he had been in his cradle.

Weeks went on with doctors' appointments. It seemed like they never ended. We eventually were spaced out with doctors' appointments. First weekly, then every other week, then every 3 weeks etc. We were also trying to reschedule an eye doctor appointment for an ERG, but due to the earthquake the machine was broken and they were waiting for a part. It was not until May 94 when we were able to take that test. That is the one test they were awaiting for to give the final diagnosis of Joubert Syndrome. I remember Mike and me taking Joey for this test not knowing what exactly it was. When I saw the things they place on the eyeball with wires I started to cry. How could they do this to a child so small? We did the test and got the results that the ERG was fine. We met with the Geneticist and he gave the final diagnosis of Joubert Syndrome. He gave us a little bit of information about the syndrome but we wanted to know anything and everything about this syndrome.

I do not remember how Mike heard about NORD, but he called there and got all the information regarding JS. After receiving the papers in the mail and reading them all, Mike saw that there was a list of contacts for more information listed. He saw one that said Joubert Syndrome Parents In Touch Network. He called the number and talked to Mary Van Damme. This was June 94. They were just about to have the 2nd conference in Florida that July. We were still very overwhelmed with all the information that we said we would pass this conference but attend the next.

When Joey was approximately four months old we were in touch with the Early Intervention Program. That is when Joey started therapy. The next few years were pretty good; not doing much other than therapy and taking care of our little boy.

We also decided that since we educate most of the doctors here, that we would go and see Dr. Maria once a year for Joey's neuro checkup. We do have a back up here for when there are tests to be run since Joey is on medication for seizures. Our pediatrician has been wonderful with us and always corresponds with other doctors.

We have come a long way since those first days, the days when I thought we would never leave the house, never travel, or do anything other than sit in the house. Since then, Joey has been to Hawaii twice, Chicago, Indiana, Maryland, Florida four times, Pennsylvania, Las Vegas numerous time, Laughlin, NV twice, San Francisco, and San Diego many times,

To date, Joey rolls all over the room. He will try and follow you when you walk. He is trying very hard to crawl and we are working on that in therapy. He attends the local public school that has a special education classroom. This September he will be in the second grade. He also receives therapy at school. The therapy site is right on campus. The therapist comes and takes him out of the classroom, does therapy and brings him back. He also receives speech therapy there as well.

The most exciting progress that Joey has done is say MA MA...... He started saying the mmmmmmmmm sound while in Baltimore in the summer of 2000, and during our extended vacation after the conference he was saying MA MA. What a joy that is to hear.

Joey is a very lovable little boy. We work with him every day in one way or another. There are other events that have taken place over the last 6½ years of Joey's life, but that would be an entire book on its own if I were to write everything that has taken place. I am sure most of you could say the same about your precious son or daughter.

Jimmy and Jake

At the request of a few parents I'm going to try to tell our ordeal with kidney failure.

Jimmy was five years old at the time and we had just come home from a routine check-up and had our yearly bloodwork done including a CBC (complete blood count). Shortly after getting home the pediatrician called and said not to be alarmed but Jimmy is very anemic. He started asking me some questions to try to get to the root of the anemia and when nothing seemed obvious he felt it was probably nothing and we would do a few more tests specific to anemia and "watch him". This was in Feb/March 1996, we had just moved to Wisconsin from Iowa in Sept 1995. When the boys were one and two they had their first and only kidney ultra-sounds, both normal, and since we didn't have any of the retinal problems that are supposedly associated with kidney problems, we didn't give kidneys another thought!

By May 1996 Jimmy had made no progress with his blood count and showed on one of his labs called a Retic count (measures new or immature blood cells that the bone marrow is supposed to produce) was Zero! His body wasn't producing any new red blood cells to replace old or destroyed blood cells in the body. We were then referred to a hematologist, went through a very traumatic bone-marrow biopsy and were relieved when he came back and told us that it was not leukemia or any blood disorder. Phew!!! then came the "but" since the root of the problem wasn't in the blood they ran a few more tests of the blood they did get and found that Jimmy's kidneys were failing and quite badly (very high BUN & Creatinine) and were only functioning at about fifteen to twenty percent. Kidney ultrasounds for both boys quickly revealed severe multicystic disease and labs showed Jake was on his way to kidney failure but had not progressed as far as Jimmy.

With this info in hand we were immediately referred, that day, to a nephrologist who whisked us off to see a dietician, a transplant coordinator, a dialysis nurse, a social worker, and a transplant surgeon. I remember thinking—Ok, I can deal with this—he gets a kidney transplant, we go home and go back to our "normal" (ha-ha!) life. Nothing had prepared me for what we were about to experience.

We were given a time frame of about six to twelve months before he would have to start dialysis (June '96). In August '96, we were scheduled for surgery to insert his dialysis catheter and begin peritoneal dialysis. The catheter is about six to twelve inches long inserted into the lower abdomen with the end resting inside of his abdominal cavity. We chose peritoneal dialysis because we could perform this at home with the aid of a machine that looks like a VCR and hook him up at night for 10 hours while he slept. We also started shots to replace the hormone that kidney produces to stimulate the bone marrow to produce new red blood cells. He also was placed on the donor waiting list.

In the meantime Jimmy had been placed on a Renal Diet which consists of low potassium, low phosphorus and low protein diet. Because the kidneys regulate electrolytes and minerals and when failing can't, this is attempted to be regulated with meds and supplements all of which were horrible tasting and we couldn't get Jimmy to take. One month later we were back in surgery for a surgically placed G-tube, in retrospect—a true blessing. He not only got his meds through this but we had to begin feedings. Toxins that build up in the blood cause general malaise, fatigue, decreased appetite, horrible smelling breath, alter the sense of taste to metallic, itchy skin and to top it off, the dialysis pulls protein off of the body. Jimmy was 5 years old, 36 inches long and weighed 20lbs! Thus, the feedings.

Next came the decision of who was to donate. For me it wasn't a decision: I was the one who would donate and don't you dare tell me I can't!!! My husband (the rational one in crisis) convinced me that it could not be me—I had to take care of Jimmy and we still had Jake to worry about. OK, no problem Jim, then you do it! OK, then which one of us is going to work? That's true: life goes on and bills will still keep coming not to mention if something went wrong, was it worth the risk of losing Jim or me? We decided—no. We decided we would wait for an anonymous donor from someone who had passed away unless the wait was too long for our comfort or Jimmy simply couldn't wait any longer at which point we would reevaluate our decision and go from there.

Jim was tested just in case. In the meantime, we received multiple phone calls from family members and friends demanding that they be "the one". We were overwhelmed with the love and concern but thought about it and evaluated how this would affect each one of these persons lives, thanked them and decided to stick with our original plan. Even Jimmy's special ed teacher (who loves him like her own) discussed this with her entire family who were all in agreement to allow her to donate if she was a "match"!

The waiting was more agonizing than anything I had ever imagined. Although Jimmy was somewhat better from the dialysis, we couldn't help but think—what are we going to do if he's not here tomorrow? He was so sickly and frail that I was scared to death that one morning his little body would decide he'd had enough and give in. The other day I came across a picture of him at his sickest and was literally mortified by his appearance—skin and bones, grey color and lifeless but smiling. I couldn't help but cry—tears of joy I think for escaping death.

We were then dealt a blow by our insurance company who smugly informed us that—by the way, you know you can't have Jimmy's transplant in Milwaukee, don't you? They are not an approved "center for excellence" (whatever the hell that means). So now we had to leave all the doctors and staff who had helped us this far, people we'd grown to trust with our little boy's life and who knew Jimmy the best. I don't know that up until that time I have ever felt such fury. We were given a choice between Chicago or Madison, WI, both at least a couple hours away. We chose Chicago because of Jim's parents living downtown and most of our family being from Illinois. The hospital there was oozing with knowledge and technology; however, it was an absolute dump and not at all family friendly, short of the associated Ronald McDonald house where we lived for two weeks. What a wonderful place!

I woke up Christmas Eve, 1996 crying, exhausted and scared. He had been on the list four months now, and I don't think I could wait another day. My husband and I held each other and cried together and quietly decided that if Jimmy didn't make it at least we could be at peace in knowing that this little boy was loved more than life itself and we had given him the best of everything we could afford. We also decided that if things went terribly wrong we would not keep him alive by artificial means.

My parents were in town visiting for the holidays from out of state but were traveling three hours to our home town to visit the grandparents for Christmas eve. Jim's parents were coming for dinner that evening so I regained my composure and tried to put my energy into preparing dinner. There were no gifts this year nor could I bring myself to put up the tree. This Christmas was to be about Jimmy and only Jimmy; that's all I wanted to have memory of.

The transplant coordinator called that afternoon just to see where we could be reached over the holidays in case we had travel plans—no, we'll be home with Jimmy. I was pulling the roast out of the oven around six o'clock that evening when the phone rang. I yelled for Jim to pick it up, it continued to ring so I answered to a voice asking "well, are you ready?" I curtly answered "ready for what?" (I was in no mood for games!). All I remember hearing was "we have a kidney, the donor is on the table—get down here now!" Needless to say, my heart was pounding and the next two weeks became a blur!

Jimmy did extremely well and continues to do great. We only know that his donor was a sixteen year old male who suffered some sort of traumatic death and that he was a transplant surgeon's dream. It's quite hectic for the first several months with lab work and doctors appointments several times a week which taper off over the next year.

Poor Jake was put on the back burner for nearly two years while Jimmy consumed me and needed my care but now it was time to concentrate on Jake. I did everything I could to get Jake in as good a condition as I could, demanding that a feeding tube be inserted early on so I could supplement his meals with feedings to keep his weight up and keep as much muscle mass as possible. I also started watching his diet like a hawk, limiting his potassium, phosphorus and protein and bombarding him with high calorie, high calcium foods. Kidney failure also pulls calcium right out of the bones due to absorption abnormalities. Although none of what I was doing could delay the inevitable I would at least try to keep him from feeling and looking so "sick".

Jake began his rapid decline in the spring of '98 when he was six years old. He, much like Jimmy, was given the six to twelve month time frame before dialysis would start. We again chose home dialysis which we were able to delay until November '98. In the mean time I fought the insurance company tooth and nail to allow us to have Jake transplanted here in Milwaukee. After much deliberation and contract negotiation with the hospital they agreed and we were ecstatic.

Jake's situation was a little different in that the doctors were trying to get him on "the list" and transplant him prior to needing to start dialysis because we were able to keep him in such good shape and knew about his failure early on. He went on the list Sept '98 but had to start dialysis in November right before Thanksgiving. It was another somber Christmas though somewhat easier than a couple of Christmases ago. I guess having gone through it once before and the comfort in knowing we weren't going to be so far from home helped.

Christmas came and went with no phone call and I started to get discouraged again. Then on January 11th, 1999 at two o'clock in the morning we got another "are you ready" call! This time the answer was a resounding YES! Jake received the kidney of a 42-year-old local woman who we believe was killed in an auto accident. We cased the news all morning while we waited for the surgery to take place and the statistics seemed to fit.

Jake's surgery went well, short of the kidney being a little sluggish at first and seizing in the car on the way to his follow-up appointment one week after surgery. The seizure, they believe, was caused by one of the anti-rejection med levels being too high. It was adjusted and he only had one other seizure shortly after the first and has not had any since. Jake, like Jimmy, is doing fantastic and I'm told are very lucky that neither one has ever suffered a rejection episode which is not that uncommon. They are both on medication for life and will probably have to be re-transplanted sometime in the future. Kidney transplants last on average fifteen to twenty years.

I have not written or contacted the donor families yet. I have tried several times to sit down and compose a letter but nothing I ever write seems worthy enough for the gifts we have been given. I cry over the frustration—how do you ever thank someone for saving your child's life in the midst of dealing with their own tragedy? I'm determined to get this done because I want these families to know that their gift will never be taken for granted. We are downright neurotic when it comes to giving the boys their meds, going to appointments and getting their labs done. Our boys will never be allowed to forget what they have been given.

The signs and symptoms of kidney failure do not show up until late in the game. There are some subtle signs such as decreased appetite, fatigue and general malaise early in failure but are difficult to spot especially when your child can't talk let alone explain to you how they feel. This is why I'm such a strong advocate of the labwork. Part of being a nurse is putting the pieces of a puzzle together so that you can present the whole picture to the doctor. The labs are a very big piece of that puzzle—they're like the ruler for measuring the percentage of kidney functioning and estimating how long that kidney will last or how well or not well the kidney is functioning. The ultrasound will show you a picture of the structure of the kidney but it tells you nothing about how well the kidney is functioning. Don't get too hung up on the ultrasound! If it's abnormal—get the labs. If the labs are normal—don't worry for now just stay on top of it with the labs every six to twelve months. The labs helped me cope with Jake's failure and gave me time to prepare to deal with what would lie ahead for him. There are specific markers in the labs that tell you when it's time to start meds, when to start dialysis, and when you're eligible for the transplant list amongst other things that the doctors watch for.

Aaron

Well, where do I begin? I guess at the very beginning. My husband and I got married in November of 1994.

Five weeks after our marriage I became pregnant with our first child. A mixture of emotions filled us both as we were still really getting to know each other, finding security emotionally and financially as we began our new life together, as all new couples must do. Although I was excited, surprised, and scared all at the same time, happiness dominated over all of these. I've always loved children and knew I wanted a family of my own someday and often envisioned what it would be like to get married and be a wife and eventually a mommy! My pregnancy was very smooth for the first two trimesters and then I went into preterm labor at six months. So, needless to say, the next three months were difficult but Adam was full term, taken only nine days early. He was, and always has been, very healthy and happy.

On Adam's second birthday, I had a miscarriage. This was a big shock as I had taken a pregnancy test and it was negative. We weren't trying for another baby yet and I had had no clues that I was pregnant. I was probably about five to six weeks along. It was fairly painless physically as it ended up being a basically normal cycle for me. It would have been much more difficult emotionally had I known I was pregnant all that time.

Aaron's story really begins May of 1998. We were ready to start thinking about having a little brother or sister for Adam. Between three and four years seemed to be a good distance between children for us, so we tried and "succeeded" the first time. This would make the kids about 3½ years apart, and that sounded great to me! Again, the pregnancy was smooth and I felt great. The day came for the ultrasound where you can determine the gender if the baby turns to the right during the procedure. Well, Aaron turned right, and there was no question as to whether the baby would be named Erin or Aaron. Adam would have a brother! We were really excited and Adam loved the idea of a new baby brother.

It was the next fifteen to twenty minutes that I remember vividly as being the beginning of this "new and unexpected journey." The sonographer, after determining the sex and checking the entire body, went back to his head where she spent several minutes just looking... and looking. I didn't ask any questions right then so as not disturb her but I was inwardly disturbed, wondering what she was concerned about to spend that much time there. I finally did ask and she said that it looked to her like there was a bigger than normal space for fluid in the third and/or fourth ventricles of his brain. She was very calm about it and did not disturb us unduly but felt it necessary for us to see a specialist whenever it could be scheduled. She told us that we'd need to be seen by Dr. J. as he was one of the best sonographers around. That made me feel good in the midst of this panic. The doctor was not in that particular day, so we made an appointment which I remember being several days later. They were LONG days for me to say the least!

We went for out first visit to Dr.J. I felt as though we "connected" immediately in the sense of his caring and completely ethical nature. I felt very comfortable talking with him, and of course respected his expertise. He did a scan and thought Aaron's condition involved a missing vermis in the cerebellum. He said that he actually didn't see it at all, which medically is called vermis agenesis. He said there was no real way to know if part of it might actually be there but he "just didn't see it." The sonographer who did the original scan worked with Dr. J and agreed with his thoughts. Vermis agenesis as an isolated thing is extremely rare, and Dr. J did a search on his computer that day and found a few articles with very little information about vermis agenesis. Of course my mind was racing a million miles a minute but I was able to compose myself. Actually I was trying to convince myself that this must be wrong, and that "part" was really there. Then reality would hit and I knew that a specialist wouldn't say something like this if he didn't feel there was a good possibility that he was correct. He did preface everything by saying that this is what he thought the situation was. We saw him a couple of other times and then he referred us to another doctor, an O.B. specialist in the same city, Dr. S.

Dr. S was the doctor who ended up delivering Aaron. From the time we visited him, he sort of took control of our "case" and we only saw Dr. J another time or two. The most stressful part of the scans the two doctors were doing is that they weren't seeing the same thing! We knew about the excess fluid in the ventricles but Dr. J. didn't see the cerebellar vermis and Dr. S didn't think there was a corpus colossum. That really shocked me and I knew that I couldn't get too out of control about my frustration, so I really prayed a lot about it and decided that maybe they were both wrong and both parts were there! I chose to try to only be concerned with the fluid, which was something that could be seen and measured. The doctors never came to an agreement before Aaron's birth.

We saw Dr. S for a regular visit somewhere about the middle of January. Aaron was due on February 13th, so it took me a little by surprise when he decided to do the section in about a week, on the 26th. There were concerns about the strength of the placenta, the umbilical cord was "unhealthy", and my fluid was low, as was the case in the first pregnancy. We knew the delivery would be c-section because we wanted the head protected and also, he ended up being breech. So, all things considered, we'd let Aaron grow and develop as much as Dr. S. felt was safe for him, and then go ahead and take him a few weeks early.

So, the big day has arrived. The surgery was scheduled for 8:00 am, so we had to leave in time to be there by 6:30. It was VERY cold, but no bad weather thank goodness! We got there, checked in, and went back to start the prep. Todd was right there with me and though he has a weak stomach in most cases, he did wonderfully. He even got great pictures of him being born. I was really proud for his strong stomach! I guess when it's your own son it's different, huh! I remember feeling the tightness and feeling myself being pulled back and forth a bit and knew Aaron would soon see us for the first time. My heart smiled and cried as I heard his first very faint cry. After a few minutes I got to kiss him and hold him before they took him to NICU. They wanted to take precautions since we really did not know what the situation would be yet. He was taken to the regular nursery later that day as the neurosurgeon and doctors were "unimpressed" as far as any real problems.

He had a CT scan done at two days of age. I vividly remember listening to Dr. A , the neurosurgeon telling us that both parts of his brain in question were there, and that if this were his child, he "wouldn't fret." He said we'd probably want to have a MRI done at about a year just for curiosity sake. He said that he wasn't telling us that everything was exactly normal, but nothing to worry excessively about. I was so relieved and really couldn't believe that both parts were really there. But who was I to argue. I was thrilled that we were taking home a healthy baby!

We stayed an extra day in the hospital due to feeding difficulties he was having. He didn't seem interested in eating at all. He wouldn't latch on to nurse, and when he did, the high roof in his mouth would cause the suction to break and he'd get frustrated and then not try at all. Another aspect is that it took ten days for my milk to come in. So, I was pumping only colostrum and he was taking maybe 10 cc at a time! He lost significant weight and the pediatrician (and I) wanted us to stay and resolve the feeding issue before he was taken home. We had to start supplementing with formula immediately (which disappointed me, but I knew we really didn't have a choice). He went from 6 lbs. 9½ oz down to 5 lbs. 13 oz in those two to three days. He was able to suck better on the small bottles that hold 30 cc. He was taking 30 cc at a time by the time we left. He gained back enough that the doctor felt OK about letting us take Aaron home.

We had several visits to our pediatrician in our hometown for weight checks. He was really tiny, and wasn't gaining very quickly. I remember getting a call from our pediatrician, Dr. P, that she wanted to have a chromosome study done and to be seen by a geneticist. There were things about Aaron, that were "different" from the start, and she really felt that it warranted being seen by a specialist. The things we saw as different were his big toes being much bigger and wider relative to "fitting with" the other toes. When I first saw his toes, I just thought, "Well, he was three weeks early - maybe he's just not quite "done" yet!"

The lactation consultant in the hospital told us that Aaron had a really high palate which certainly contributing to his difficulty in suckling and swallowing. Also, since just hours after birth, he had what the pediatrician at the hospital called a little whimper which he said he'd never seen before like that. Aaron literally vocalized with every breath and the breaths were very rapid. I about hyperventilated just listening to him. We were really concerned but all of the doctors would just say "It's newborn tachypnea and he'll outgrow it." I never bought that and knew in my heart that there was something more to it, especially when he got to be eight months old and it was still there, though much better. But still, he was no longer considered a newborn.

We saw the geneticist on February 15th, at about the age of 3 weeks, and he mentioned Rubinstein Taybi Syndrome to us. I was really trying to concentrate and listen to what he was saying even though I was dying inside to think there was really something wrong with Aaron. After all, we left the hospital thinking all was just fine. I asked again the name of the syndrome and made a concerted mental effort to remember that name—Rubinstein Taybi. He told us it was very rare. He said that was what he thought Aaron had and that although he had some of the characteristics, there were many he didn't have. When I read about RTS later, I just thought that anything Aaron didn't have, or didn't experience, was just an indication that he was a "mild" case. So from February on, I found all of the information I could about RTS.

The day I first read about the syndrome is etched into my memory. My mom had looked up RTS on the Internet, and after Aaron was down for a nap, I went and read about it. My heart literally tore apart as I sat there and read about these kids and what is known about this syndrome. The first time I read the words mentally retarded, I got numb all over. From that point, and for about two weeks following, I experienced what I know was my "grieving period" and coming to terms with reality. I didn't want to get upset in front of my mom, so I acted like I needed to go to the mall and pick up something. I drove straight out to the school where Todd worked and just prayed that he was on campus and in his office. Well, he wasn't in his office and in fact not even on campus. A couple of people talked to me but I honestly don't remember what they said or asked. I was trying so desperately to maintain control and not break down right there. One of the secretaries told me he was gone and she didn't know when he'd be back. I needed to talk to him so badly. I got back in the car and decided to drive awhile. About a half mile down the road, I saw him heading back toward school. I turned around and went back to catch up with him.

He was waiting on me and got in the car. I was so glad I didn't miss him. He didn't have any idea what was wrong. I broke down, and told him that I'd read details about RTS and this really looks like what Aaron had. I knew specifics about IQ potential, average height, ability to live independently, and most likely inability to have children. I was a basket case to say the least. Todd was really seemingly calm about things and told me that "even if Aaron couldn't give us grandchildren, he'll give us many other things". We talked about thirty minutes and then I went back home after I felt composed enough. Little did I know that Todd really went through a tough time mentally about this, too, but felt like he needed to remain all right for my sake so kept it to himself. I was glad when he finally opened up, though it took him a little while to totally come to terms with it himself, if that has even fully happened yet. Does it ever REALLY happen?

That was the beginning of a full two-week period that I was emotionally out of control. Aaron was the most precious little boy and I couldn't imagine him not perfect in every way and that he wouldn't have the most normal and happy life like Adam, our other son. I felt bad about being so engrossed in Aaron and wanted and needed to spend quality time with Adam. He really adjusted wonderfully to his new brother. To this day, he has never seemed jealous or "mistreated" when I've had to spend time feeding or caring for Aaron. It was amazing how my outlook seemed to change after that two weeks. It didn't and doesn't change the pain at the core of my heart for the fact that Aaron won't experience life the same way Adam or any other "normal" child will. But, I no longer feel sorry for myself or for Aaron.

I owe this feeling of "peace" to the fact that I gave this totally to God and I know everything will be all right. He is much more in control than I could even think I am. It was strange how at that two-week period, I just felt this inner peace that I've never felt before and I've never gone back to that feeling of total helplessness and hurt. One other thing that helped me was the parent support list I found on the Internet. There are almost 400 families in this group of families with children of all ages affected by RTS. That was literally my saving grace during this time of realization and coming to terms with all of this. It was a family to go to with questions, concerns, for advice—anything you wanted to say or ask, and they were there to respond and encourage me every step of the way.

Aaron was the youngest one at the time we got on the list. So many of the things that were discussed, I could shake my head and say yes, that's Aaron. But there were many things that weren't like Aaron. Things like: severe constipation, needing g-tubes because of such severe feeding difficulties, undescended testicles, head circumference in the 5th percentile (Aaron's has been in the 95th % since birth), and the "look" that these kids have. Aaron did NOT look like them. Again, I just thought, well this is just the mildness of his case and we're really lucky. We saw the geneticist again, and his partner who actually saw Aaron, again said that RTS did look like what Aaron had. I didn't expect him to say otherwise.

By now it was September. We had moved to Georgetown, KY, just outside Lexington. We knew about the geneticist here at the University and what good hands Aaron would be in. That made me feel great. We saw him one day in mid-September and he informed us that he did not think Aaron had RTS. In fact if RTS had not been mentioned, he never would have considered it as a possibility! No telling how big my eyes got on that one. I just couldn't believe it. At the same time, it answered a lot of my questions about why no one identified with his breathing; fluid in the ventricles of his brain; testicles that were descended; bigger—not smaller—head; and many other things. He said he thought Aaron had Joubert Syndrome and asked if I'd ever heard of it. I told him yes, but didn't know where or what it was. He told us a little about it and also that it was very rare—four times as rare as RTS! I found out that the literature has about 200 known cases. So, I was literally back to square one as far as my knowledge about the syndrome and where to go from here as far as tests to be done and what potential medical problems to rule out.

The doctor told us that to confirm Joubert, we'd need to have a MRI done, because part or all of the vermis must be missing. I immediately thought of Dr. J. but knew that Aaron was not missing any parts as far as the CT scan at birth was concerned. We scheduled the MRI and had it done on November 3rd. What I really felt like had happened is that they didn't look closely enough or couldn't see well enough on the CT scan and maybe missed that fact that a portion of the vermis was really missing. We did find out the results that day.

We had an appointment about three hours after the MRI with the ophthalmologist who was to do eye surgery on Aaron the next morning, Nov. 4th. He walked down to radiology and saw the images and talked to the technician himself. He came back into the room, and told us that Aaron seemed to be a "classic textbook case of Joubert Syndrome." First question from me was, "What about the vermis?" He said, "Total agenesis." I had to have him repeat that, as I couldn't believe what I was hearing—TOTAL AGENESIS? I then realized that Dr. J's instincts from the very beginning were right on the mark. That didn't change the fact of his probable diagnosis anyway, but what had they seen on the CT scan? Had they literally "seen something" that wasn't, and never had, been there? That's still a mystery to me.

We decided to postpone the surgery because of his breathing (tachynea/apnea) which had gotten better but was definitely still there. There are serious concerns about administering anesthesia and the effect that it may have on his already abnormal breathing patterns. Joubert

Syndrome might have its own form of apnea. He never stops for more than seven or eight seconds at a time; thus it's not apnea in the true medical sense, (which I found is for fifteen seconds or longer! That would really scare me!) He's never turned blue or reacted in a scared or urgent way about beginning breathing again. I would be very much more insistent on addressing the breathing with apnea monitoring or in other ways if that were the case.

I stay at home with the boys and I wouldn't trade this job for anything in the world. Aaron has therapy four times a week. He's had early intervention since about two months of age. The misdiagnosis didn't in any way change what we've done as far as his intervention or his ability to qualify for such services. It's just been quite a roller coaster. I also have really tried not to lose focus of what a happy and healthy baby Aaron is. He has to be one of the most happy, content babies I've ever seen. Yes, he has his moments, but most cries are very purposeful. He is quite delayed with his milestones due to his low muscle tone. He has all of the cardinal symptoms of Joubert Syndrome. 1) Low muscle tone 2) Vermal agenesis 3) Excessive fluid in the 4th ventricle of the brain 4) Abnormal eye and tongue movements. and 5) breathing abnormality.

He can't sit up independently, get on all fours, crawl, etc. He does roll all around the room. He's holding his head up a lot better for several seconds at a time while on his tummy. There is so much about the future that is unknown. We just take things one day at a time, and enjoy each day for what it is—a gift. I must educate myself as much as possible for Aaron's best interest. From what I hear, much of the medical community is just now really becoming aware of this syndrome. It was discovered in 1969, but due to low numbers, follow-up studies in many cases just aren't there. It's just not common at all.

Aaron's big smiles and sweet nature make it so easy for me to be happy and content with reality, though it's not easy, and will never be "normal." I also have thought lately how I must treasure these first couple of years, because I know that the time when walking, talking, potty training and all of the other milestones that come with age—are unknown for Aaron. Again, I don't feel sorry for him anymore; I must be strong for him and experience his milestones with him on his time clock. He wouldn't want me to feel sorry for him. He has taught me so many lessons about life already. He is a definite light in our lives. There is a connection with him that I can't explain. Any parent can identify, but a special needs child certainly puts a new twist on that. He loves his big brother and Adam surely adores him.

One other piece of information about Joubert Syndrome, and I guess the most surprising thing we've found out, is that it's an auto-recessive gene that was passed to him by both myself and my husband. We did the math in the geneticist's office last week. Taking two people randomly who are married, there is a one in 275,000 chance that Joubert Syndrome would show itself. Todd and I were both carriers from one side of both parents. The gene hasn't been identified, so there's no way to know where it came from and how many generations it has been passed before this one in four chance happened with Aaron. Interesting and crazy, huh??!??

This has become longer than I anticipated but I guess that's the way it usually is when you're "telling a story from the beginning." I do realize that life is a journey filled with highs, lows and everything in between. I honestly believe that because of the difficulties Aaron might face in the future, all of the highs in his life, big or small, will be even greater and more fulfilling for all of us who experience them with him. I cannot imagine my life without him and anyone that has the privilege of coming in contact with him will be forever blessed. All children are truly gifts from God and our boys have enriched our lives beyond words in these first five short years. God is good.

Aimee and Lige

Aimee's story began October 20, 1988. She weighed eight pounds. She was born to Lige and Tammy in Louisiana. Aimee is the third child in the family. She had many difficulties at birth. She was born blue with no reactions to stimulation at all. We were told she suffered from anoxia, lack of oxygen to the brain. After a little while, we noticed she wasn't looking at us. At three weeks old, her head began shaking from side to side at all times except sleep. We rushed her to the hospital and that was when our journey began: seeing one doctor after another, week after week, day after day. When she visited the Louisiana Lions Eye Center, a total of ten doctors came to see her in one day. They could not believe all the different eye abnormalities she had. We were told she was blind. At three months old, a pediatric neurologist told us she would never be or do anything. She said we should start saving our money for a wheelchair—we would need it. We were not given much hope for her future. We immediately started with early intervention and physical and occupational therapies. She was very tactiile defensive. She had such a high, narrow palette that she could not suck a bottle correctly. She stayed really small for a long time. She has ataxic cerebral palsy, is visually impaired, is developmentally delayed and is still tactile defensive. She is mildly mentally deficient and has lots of trouble with balance. She cannot ride a two wheel bike which bothers her a great deal. She wants to be like the other kids and do as they do. She reads and writes Braille. She attends school at the Louisiana school for the Visually Impaired. She has many friends and is very social.

Aimee loves to sing and dance. She sat up at eighteen months old and she walked at four years old with a walker. She now walks and runs. She now has speech, OT, PT, Orientation and Mobility, Adaptive Physical Education, Living Skills and piano lessons. She loves to cook and help with the work. She enjoys camping, swimming and playing with her cats. She's crazy about Britney Spears, Barbies, and of course, Sailor Moon! She has an older sister named Jessica and an older brother Marshal. She had a little sister named Gracie who passed away in 1997. She did not have Joubert Syndrome.

Aimee now has a little brother with Joubert Syndrome. His name is Lige. Aimee was recently diagnosed with JS after the baby was born. We were so glad to finally have a diagnosis.

We were blessed with baby Lige on June 25, 1999. He weighed 6 lbs, 15½ oz. at birth even though he was six weeks early. During pregnancy, we were told he would possibly have Dandy-Walker Malformation (a fluid filled cyst on the brain). He could not keep his body temperature up, he kept losing weight and he could not get his suck/breathe/swallow together. He also had apnea. He stayed in NICU for ten days. At two weeks old, he still would not gain weight. When we brought him home from the NICU, he weighed 6 lbs, 7 oz. He was put back in the hospital for "failure to thrive" mostly as he was throwing up all he drank. He came home again, this time on an apnea monitor—what a pain that was! He has been in and out of the hospital for hernia surgery, tubes in ears, pneumonia, sleep studies and PH Probe tests. He is now doing well.

He is full of joy! He is just beginning to roll over and hold his head up. He is visually impaired but we don't know how much yet. He is beginning to try to speak by babbling "bye bye". We are proud that God felt that we were worthy to have all of our children. It is a challenge every day, but we would not trade it for any other kind of life. these children make us special, too! We hope only the best for their futures. Now matter what kind of child you consider yourself to have, just remember each one is a perfect gift from God.

Luise

Judi's mom

A faith journey is a lifelong process. Mine continues. Without one's awareness, this journey begins as a baby and progresses stage by stage.

My first conscious awareness of faith came as a young

adult with the birth of our first child. My faith was weak and certainly out of focus! Believe in God, go to church, try to do right as Jesus taught, and life goes according to plan. And I had a plan....

From near the onset of my first pregnancy I had the feeling that all was not well, but medically everything progresses satisfactorily. Still the feeling persisted. In September 1970, I was awakened in the night by a beautiful, peaceful, loving voice telling me my baby would be a boy born with hydrocephalus. The voice vanished; I felt puzzled and worried, but shared the experience with no one. Soon thereafter medical problems began, ending with my hospitalization and then at home in bed for the final two months of the pregnancy. In December 1970, delivery day came, inducing labour failed, an emergency C-section followed, a boy with severe hydrocephalus and other birth anomalies was born and I was devastated! My plan!

Emotional upheaval, denial, and caring for him intertwined, plus anger and bitterness toward God, all coloured by exhaustion of body and soul made for tumultuous weeks! How could a loving God whom I had tried to serve do this? to me? to a baby??? Six months later our Timothy died! Why would God do this when we really wanted children?—yes, four healthy, strong, intelligent children! Question upon question, usually self-directed—why me?

I was searching, reading, and continued actively in our church. Two ladies at our church were caring and supportive and even visited us regularly. My parents were pillars of love and support. However, most people, some family and friends included, chose to distance themselves because the situation made them "feel bad" or inadequate.

Life continued. Then in February 1972, that same beautiful, peaceful, loving voice again spoke during the night. The message: a girl who would live with a December 16th date given. Pregnancy soon followed.

Judi was born on December 6th, a girl who did not breathe spontaneously, had extra and webbed great toes and complete ptosis of her right eye. As time progressed, development was slow, special needs obvious. My emotional state was in chaos: likewise, my spiritual life. But God never moved! He was there, always protecting and guiding. Many times there seemed no way, but a new path was lit! Through the years, by God's constant love and presence, the fellowship of believers, personal prayer and study, my faith has grown and continues to be polished to this day!

I now have inner peace and abiding joy. Outward circumstances of many different origins are still troublesome and disappointing, but I know that God is in control and will guide, direct, and make a way if I put my faith and trust in Him. A personal, constant closeness with God and Jesus truly sets me free.

Through the years I've come to feel that God does not choose someone to have disabilities, accidents and the like or to be parent of such a special person. However, God allows these things to happen. The universe and all the laws concerning its rhythms are set. Genetically some combinations are faulty. God could step in and prevent the result. However, many times the natural process is allowed to proceed.

With God's help, struggles, questions, and sorrows build one to a full being capable of compassion, empathy, and understanding toward others. Valleys and mountain tops! One leads to and enhances the other! God's grace, care, and love is given new every morning. Plug into the power source to go through the joys and challenges of each day. Sometimes God is better glorified by patient endurance and inner joy in the face of challenge.

Sharie

mom to Spencer, Christopher and Jason

Our family has been blessed with four beautiful children. Spencer Jeffrey born October 2, 1982, Melissa Daphney born June 12, 1984, Christopher Scott born June 20, 1987, and Jason David born July 17, 1989. The three boys have Joubert Syndrome. We have been privileged to know and love each of our children with their individual talents, personalities, and strengths.

Our journey began while I was attending High school, my Junior year in Lyman, Wyoming. Lyman is a very small town. In 1979 there was only one gymnasium and one cafeteria for all of the grade levels to share. During the high school lunch period time, the special needs children, with their aids, would be eating in the cafeteria too.

There was one little boy in particular. He had difficulty with swallowing and it bothered me to look at him. Every bite that was put into his mouth would come back out all over. It made lunch less appetizing if I was sitting where I could see this little boy eat.

The fact that I felt uncomfortable around children who had special needs bothered me. I had felt for years that I would one day give birth to my own handicapped child. How was I going to love my own child when I felt fear and disgust being near other special needs children? One night, I pondered this question. I prayed and asked God to help me. It was during that prayer that I heard a small child's voice speak "Mother". I was surprised and in disbelief of what I had just heard. But I soon drifted off to sleep.

The next morning I awoke with the same question still on my mind. How could I be the mother of a handicapped child if I couldn't stand to be around children like that? I got up and took the bus to school. Still feeling perplexed by this dilemma I went to my first period class which was gym. I knew it would be early enough that I would be alone so I went into the girls' locker room and knelt down to pray. Again, I asked God how I could be a mother to a special needs child if I could not stand to be around them.

Just then I heard someone walking out of the showers. Startled, I felt embarrassed. I thought I had been alone. I quickly got to my feet just in time to see a little girl with Down Syndrome walking towards me from out of the showers. At first I thought it was a vision of a future child, but when she came close enough I could see she was real. I reached out to touch her and just as I did I was filled with a love for her that I never felt before. I walked her over to the middle school where the special education children met. I found out that her mother was the new special education teacher, Mrs. Bradshaw, and I found out how I could help out with these children. I started working with Mrs. Bradshaw whenever time would allow. I grew to love each one of these children including Brent who was the adorable little boy with feeding issues.

When Spencer was born, he had irregular rapid breathing and they placed him in the ICU. He remained there for eight days. While there Spencer was jaundiced, had some head swelling, still had this rapid breathing with periodic times when he would stop breathing. They did a spinal tap and said he had a Subaracnoid Hemorrhage. When we took him home there were still concerns about his head swelling and a possible need for a shunt. They also told us that there was a possibility that Spencer might not make it. We felt confident that Spencer would live and that he was the special needs child that I heard call out to me one night years ago as a teenager.

There were a lot of births in our church community right around the same time Spencer was born. At Christmas, our church had a live nativity. They chose another little baby boy to play Jesus. As I was looking over this baby Jesus, I noticed that this little baby was looking back straight into my eyes. That was when I knew something was wrong with Spencer's eye sight. Spencer's eyes roamed around in their sockets and were very red and watery all the time.

We got an appointment at the University of Utah with a Dr. J. She was a specialist with children. She did an ERG on Spencer and told us that he had Cortical blindness with light perception only. She went on to say that he would never attend a normal school nor drive a car. Dr. J encouraged us to read a book called *Can't Your Child See?* I felt stunned and sick inside. I never thought that my baby would be blind. As the doors shut to the elevator I began to cry. Bart my husband jumped all over me saying, "Don't you cry." I said, "How dare you tell me not to cry, my baby will never see my face!" Bart said, "Yes, he will. He'll be fine". It has been this positive attitude that Bart had from the beginning that has pulled our family through. When we got home we put Christmas lights all around the top of Spencer's crib. We then put Christmas lights all over the house, wherever we usually placed his infant seat. If Spencer had light perception only, we were going to use this strength and build on it.

We next held a special prayer and fast with the members in our church and at the end of the fast time Bart's father Reed who was the bishop of our church at the time, gave Spencer a special blessing by the power of the Holy Melchizedek Priesthood, which restored Spencer's eye sight. Five months later when we returned to Dr. J's office she was shocked to see the change in Spencer's eye sight.

After nursing for a year the next hurdle was Spencer's difficulty with swallowing baby food. He looked in fact very much like that little boy Brent that I grew to love so much in high school. Spencer had a huge protruding tongue that hung out most of the time. All the food that I tried to get into his mouth came back out in his saliva. I was afraid that he would starve to death. One morning after trying again to get some baby food down Spencer, I knelt down in exasperation and pleaded our cause before the Lord. I told him I knew He could heal Spencer so that he could in fact swallow. After the prayer, I tried feeding him again and my prayer was heard. Spencer could swallow.

Spencer's development was severely delayed. He was like a new born infant the whole first year of life. Spencer did not even have the normal abilities of making a fist, or sucking on his fingers. His little arms were too weak to raise his hands up to his mouth. Nor did he do the cute stretching of his little arms above his head as most little infants do. He was like a little limp rag doll. I did three hours of therapy with Spencer every day. I put together my own schedule of exercises from watching the OT and PT that I took him to see twice a week at the Child Development center. I felt that some how my body had caused him to be this way and I had to do every thing in my power to heal him. It was not until years later that a therapist told me that I could not heal my son's muscle tone by doing therapy with them. She relieved a huge heavy burden from my shoulders. Spencer progressed very slowly by his second birthday. He still had not had a lot of his firsts that were normally recorded by parents in baby books. He eventually learned to sit slouched over and from there began to scoot on his bottom. He learned to clap his feet long before he was ever able to clap his hands. I encouraged four point rocking in our therapy sessions but Spencer never learned to crawl normally until years later.

Melissa was born twenty months later. She was a joy. My only regret was not being able to enjoy her more. Her needs did not compare to that of Spencer's so she sat content most of the time in her infant chair. She grew up in the shadow of Spencer's doctor appointments and therapy sessions.

Christopher was born three years later. The pregnancy and birth went with out a hitch. We truly thought Christopher was normal. No sticking out of the tongue, no irregular or rapid breathing, no nystagmus. He could grasp your finger but it was not real firm. His head control was still a little wobbly but better than that of Spencer's. Our PT would come out to the house for Spencer and kept asking if I wanted her to take a look at Christopher but I would tell her no since he was fine!

One evening while I sat at the back of the chapel nursing Christopher in a church meeting for women only, a messenger came to me. I did not see anyone but a voice, that of a female, told me that I was going to have another special needs child. I felt peace with this message and was not alarmed. But I also thought to myself that I was glad we had Christopher and I was going to really enjoy him. Then, days later while I was at a baby shower holding Christopher, a woman sitting next to me announced to the whole group, "Christopher is not focusing with his eyes." I felt mortified and I hated this woman who had suddenly made my baby boy handicapped.

We got Christopher's eye sight tested and found out that he had circular nystagmus not the usual back and forth nystagmus that Spencer had. He also had a coloboma in his right eye just like Spencer had and he was also developmentally delayed. At eleven months of age we started Christopher in the Early Intervention program in Massachusetts, where we had moved to before Christopher was born. I started doing the therapy at home that I had previously done with Spencer and continued to work with Spencer as well. However, Spencer was now in a full day school program.

Christopher's disposition was a very pleasant one as a baby. He was happy all the time and would smile and laugh as long as I did not try to do any therapy with his body. He would have been content to sit in a wheel chair all of his life and smile at everyone that passed by. He appeared to be in his own world at times, almost as if he would phase out, not like seizures, but more like autism. After the age of two, as soon as he had the muscle control, he would rock in his seat a great deal. He did not have the swallowing issues that Christopher had had. He had a normal size tongue. He was very pleasant and very social with his Chinese sounding chatter. He also had adorable blond ringlets all over his head that grew into long banana curls down his back that I swore I would not cut until he began to walk. Christopher's development was much slower than Spencer's. He was basically content to just sit back and enjoy life. Each therapy session was painful and emotional for him. He did however progress as Spencer did to sitting and to scooting on his bottom. Christopher finally began to walk around three and a half years old.

Jason was born two years after Christopher. Jason was a surprise baby. We had hoped to have another baby girl and was very disappointed when the ultrasound said it was a boy. I was certain since it was a boy, something would be wrong with him. I was afraid that my body did not like boys. (I had been dealing with issues of abuse with male perpetrators.) I got Toxemia at the end of the pregnancy as I had with Spencer's pregnancy. They put me in the hospital on full bed rest the week before he was delivered. During one of the stress tests that they did periodically to make sure the baby was okay, it sounded like I could hear Jason crying inside the womb. I wanted to get him out. I felt that my body was hurting him somehow. When Jason was born, he had the same breathing difficulties we had seen in Spencer. He was put in the ICU. Jason and I both stayed a week longer in the hospital.

When we brought him home, he came home with a staph infection on his leg that some nurse had passed to him from another patient. I kept asking the pediatrician if Jason had the same thing as his brothers. Even though there was no title for it, I knew that he did. The pediatrician did not want to give him a negative title until he was sure. After about eight months of no progress, the pediatrician agreed that Jason, too, was developmentally delayed. Jason was a very difficult baby. He cried the full first year of his life. He was very hard to console. He had reflux problems and was put on Reglin before I would nurse him. We also found that he was almost completely deaf in one ear and had little hearing in the other. He had several sets of tubes as did his brothers. The ear infections however did not stop until the ENT removed his adenoids. Jason was in so much pain that he would pull clumps of hair out of his head. We had to keep his head shaved. He would also pull and scratch at his ears so much that he often cut his ears or face with his finger nails and it seemed even if we removed them completely, he would still be able to cut his face and ears with his nails. Jason's progress was even slower than Christopher's. He did not walk until he was nearly five years of age. He was also diagnosed with failure to thrive and we gave him prescription shakes to help keep his weight up.

By this time, I had two little boys who were not mobile, and who were dead weight to carry. They both were still in need of being fed all of their meals and dressed completely. Spencer was also still in need of feeding assistance and dressing as well. We were blessed to have Dottie, a home health aid join our family and she was another true answer to prayer. She served our family for 10 years. She was not only a help with the personal care of all the boys, she helped me plan meals, do school clothes shopping and even clean the house. Every holiday we would get together with Dottie and Joe and Dottie's parents Dorothy and Edward. Dottie was not able to have children of her own and she considered our children to be her very own grandchildren. Nana and Papa N did the same.

January 1998 was when we first heard of Joubert Syndrome. Spencer woke up one morning unable to move his right arm. He was sixteen and half years old. We took him to the Children's Hospital in Boston and there they scheduled many tests. It was after a MRI that we found out that his missing vermis meant that he had the Joubert Syndrome. Spencer regained the use of his right arm in time and it was determined that it was a virus that caused his the temporary nerve damage to his right arm. We now had a diagnosis to go by. I looked Joubert up on the Internet and found the Joubert Syndrome Foundation. I was sent a packet of information on the syndrome and felt so overwhelmed that I stuck it back on a shelf for a time.

It was not until December of 1999 that we took Jason and Christopher into the Children's hospital to have an MRI done on them so that they too could be properly diagnosed. It was early in the morning that I gathered Spencer, Melissa and Edie (a friend that was staying with us) together to kneel in prayer to petition God for help with Jason and Christopher. With sixteen years of experience under our belt I knew better than to tell any of the boys before hand what was going to happen because any change from the regular schedule would knock them out of sorts. I led our family in prayer since Bart had already left for work. I asked God to help Jason and Christopher to understand why this test was necessary and to bless that it would not be traumatic for them. They were going to have to get an IV placed in their arms to be helped to sleep so that they would be still during the

MRI. I was also concerned that since they would not be able to have breakfast before they left, they would be upset. Then after the prayer, we woke Jason and Christopher up, quickly dressed them and led them directly out to the car. Christopher was the first to ask us where we were going and why. I told him we were going to the Children's hospital to take pictures of his and Jason's brain to see if there was anything wrong. Christopher said, "Is that why I am dizzy?" I did not ever hear Christopher express to me before that he felt dizzy, but in fact the part of the brain that is affected, the vermis, does control balance. It felt like Christopher was blessed with a capacity to understand things as he never had before. Christopher then said why can't Jesus just heal my dizziness. I said He could if He wanted to. We got to Children's Hospital and every thing went much better then I had anticipated. They placed a numbing cream on their arms and placed a patch over it so the needle would not hurt. They told us when the boys woke up they would be grouchy and crying and out of sorts from the effects of the drug.

Christopher went first and then it was Jason's turn. Jason began to have some breathing difficulty but the nurse tilted his head back and he was fine. Next, we were in recovery with both of them. Christopher began to stir first. I went over to him to comfort him and he was very happy. He said out loud Jesus was with me. I said what do you mean? He said Jesus came and talked to me. He told me that He loved me and wanted me to be a good boy and that He would heal me. He said other things too. The nurses gathered round and were in shock to see a little boy wake up with the effects of a drug in that way. They were fascinated at his announcement of Jesus' visit and then suddenly they acted as though it was just the effects of the medicine that made him think this. But I knew in my heart that we had again received an answer to our prayers. God has been so very close with our family as we have tried to raise our four children. We do not ever leave anything to chance. With Faith in God all things are possible.

Now at almost eighteen years of age, Spencer has almost received his Eagle rank in the scout program. He still has his Emergency Preparedness Merit badge and his project which has already been approved to do. He is very compassionate to all those around him. He is a very hard worker and receives all high grades in high school. He is presently learning at his regular grade level.

Melissa was the class president of ninth grade this year. She loves drama and reaches out to all her class mates that are less fortunate or are put down by the "in crowd".

Christopher is our family comedian. He is still always smiling and happy. He is in character most of the time. His favorite new name is Majesty.

Jason loves computer programs and his Game Boy. He is a sweet loving little boy and is very pleasant to be around.

The future looks bright for us. We are living on five acres of land that is commercially zoned in which we plan to have two big green houses and farm animals with a home for special needs adults to live and work the farm to support themselves. This will not only give our boys a place to live but possibly others as well.

This is where our Journey of prayer and faith has led.

When I first approached the families involved in the Joubert Syndrome foundation with the idea of this book, I encouraged them all to submit their stories to share with the readers. I wasn't sure at that time just what the finished book would consist of so I also supplied the following questionnaire for people who preferred more structure to their story. The following section features some of the answers to that questionnaire. Most notable is Judi's answers appearing here as on the original page, written in her own hand at the age of twenty-five.

QUESTIONNAIRE: PARENT OF PERSON WITH J.S.

CHILD'S NAME (optional):
PHONE #:
GENDER:
AGE OF CONFIRMED DIAGNOSIS:
PRESENT AGE:
AGE OF FIRST "SYMPTOMS":

How did you first suspect your child had "problems"?

How did that affect you and your family? What thoughts did you have?

When did you first hear of Joubert Syndrome? How did you feel? then? now? Do you feel that you have enough information? What do you still need to know?

When someone asks you what's wrong with your child, how do you respond? what do you say?

What was the most difficult stage in your child's development for you? for your child?

What is your main concern about your child's education? What are you doing to address it? What questions do you need answered?

Is your child at a school? home? specialized centre? What is the main challenge faced by your child at this point?

QUESTIONNAIRE: PERSON WITH J.S.

NAME (optional):
PHONE #:
GENDER:
AGE OF CONFIRMED DIAGNOSIS:
PRESENT AGE:
AGE OF FIRST "SYMPTOMS":

1. What do you know about Joubert Syndrome?

2. What does it mean to you?

3. When did you first find out that you have J.S.?

4. How did you feel then? now?

5. What do you say when someone asks “what's wrong with you”?

6. What is the most difficult part of having J.S.?

7. What is your proudest achievement?

8. What would you say to someone who just found out they have J.S.?

9. Was there a point in your life that was difficult because you have J.S.?

10. How did your family react during that time?

11. Are you at school? work? home? specialized centre?

12. What is the main challenge you face at this point of your life?

13. How are you addressing it?

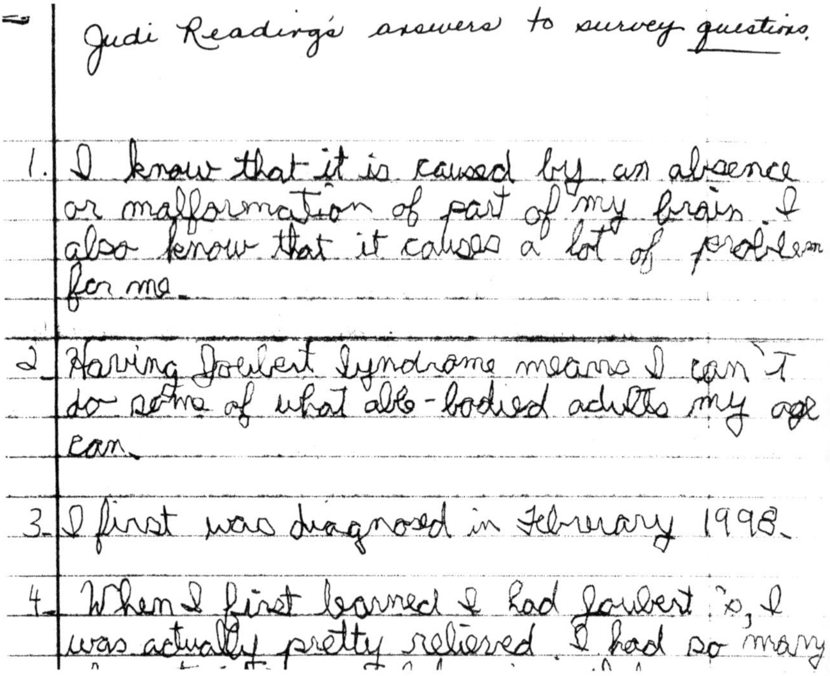
Judi Reading's answers to survey questions.

1. I know that it is caused by an absence or malformation of part of my brain. I also know that it causes a lot of problem for me.

2 Having Joubert Syndrome means I can't do some of what able-bodied adults my age can.

3. I first was diagnosed in February 1998.

4. When I first learned I had Joubert's, I was actually pretty relieved. I had so many

1. I know that it is caused by an absence or malformation of part of my brain. I also know that it causes a lot of problems for me.

2. Having Joubert Syndrome means I can't do some of what able-bodied adults my age can.

3. I first was diagnosed in February, 1998.

4. When I first learned I had Joubert's, I was actually pretty relieved. I had so many characteristics and behaviors that my previous diagnosis of cerebral palsy did not explain, but Joubert's explained all of

them! Now, after learning more information about Joubert's, I have even more explanations!

5. I say "I have Joubert's Syndrome, a rare genetic disorder" and then answer any questions they have to the best of my ability.
6. Not being understood! People think I'm lazy because I don't work and haven't finished college when in reality, I can't. The stress is too much.
7. In 1992, I won a national award for my volunteer efforts.
8. I would tell them that having Joubert Syndrome does not mean life is over. It is not something that means all they can do is vegetate somewhere and not expect to do much else. I would also tell them that it is still okay to hope and dream about the future because they do indeed have one.
9. Yes. The social aspect of school was hard. Even in high school, kids always laughed at me.
10. Mom and Dad were very sympathetic.
11. Actually, none of the three. My parents had an addition built on their home. I currently live there while continuing to do my volunteer work on Tuesday afternoons.
12. Struggling with the fact that God's plan for my life is totally opposite of what I'd like.
13. My Christian faith helps considerably. I praise Him for the blessings I do have. When times get tough, I pray for Him to give me His strength to carry on.

Colleen

Country: Ireland
Diagnosis Confirmation: 24 weeks into my pregnancy
Present Age : 4 years 8 months
Age of First Symptoms: Immediately, rapid breathing, high sodium levels(enlarged Kidneys)

- I was very fortunate as I found out before Colleen was born about her condition. Doctors painted a very black picture and we didn't expect her to live. We had time to come to terms with her condition before she arrived, so there was no panic or rejection. It was all a matter of just letting the doctors get on with their job. Naturally we were devastated. Our first born, Amy-Louise was only three years old, so this meant she was pushed from pillar to post while we spent long hours and weeks at a time in hospitals with Colleen. Amy was great, she never resented Colleen and has never ever been jealous of all the time we have to spend working with her.

- I feel we have plenty of information, although this is mainly down to my research. When Colleen was born and I asked the Neurologist for information, he said what was available was too medically technical for me but I sourced the information myself and looked up medical dictionaries to help me with phrases I didn't understand, and guess what! I figured it out anyway! I would still love a more comprehensive understanding on the life expectancy issue. Colleen doesn't really have any physical features of JS, so she looks very like her older sister, so we don't get a lot of questions when we're out, except when she gets scared and throws a tantrum. I usually just tell people that she has a very rare syndrome that leaves her both mentally and physically handicapped with other disabilities.

- I have totally accepted all Colleens disabilities, but I would dearly love it if she had some sort of intelligible speech, even if it was a form that only those close to her can understand. It would be less frustrating for her if she could let us know what she wants. At the moment her communication skills are limited to crying to let us know something is up, so its all trial and error.

- Colleen attends a wonderful special school where they cater for all her needs, ie. physio, OT, all her equipment is assessed and ordered here.

- I would love others not affected to be educated in the world of coping with a child with multiple disabilities. I felt very isolated when Colleen was born. Friends didn't call as they didn't know how to handle the situation (not true friends, I hear you say) but it was very difficult to make new friends. And took a long time. A very lonely time.

Ryan

- At birth Ryan had several problems and we were told that he needed further testing to see if we could find out what was wrong. I was heartbroken and scared to death as was our whole family. I had such thoughts as "what did I do wrong", and "what did I do or Ryan to deserve this". There was never any mention of Joubert Syndrome. Ryan was tested for cystic fibrosis, muscular dystrophy and cerebral palsy which all these tests came back negative. I was worried that I would not a strong enough person to be able to deal with a special needs child. I soon realized that Ryan was the most loving child anyone could ever ask for and that I'd do anything for him. I also wondered if there was something that I had done wrong during the pregnancy that caused this to happen to him. I blamed myself for quite awhile.

- After years of testing and simply being told that our son was just developmentally delayed we finally had an MRI done on Ryan at the age of seven and got the diagnosis of Joubert Syndrome. At first I was scared to death because even the doctor didn't know what it was or what we could do to help him. When I was over the initial shock I felt relieved because at least we now had something with a name that we could find information on and be able to help Ryan. I know that there is more for me to learn about Joubert Syndrome, but I'm feeling better about it now thanks to all the help from the Joubert Syndrome Parents in Touch Network.

- When someone asks me what is wrong with Ryan I simply tell them he has Joubert Syndrome and then I explain to them what it is and then I end by saying that I thank God everyday for bringing Ryan into our lives and making me a better and stronger person because of him. Ryan is the biggest joy and blessing in our lives and I couldn't imagine life without him.

- The most difficult stages in Ryan's development was potty training and going off to school.
- I worry that Ryan may not be getting everything he needs in school. Our school system is pretty small and I don't feel it is really up to date with such things as PT/OT, special education, etc...
- Ryan lives at home with us (father, mother and older sister who is 14 and not affected in anyway) and he is in a regular 4th grade classroom in school.
- Ryan's biggest challenge that he is facing today is his hand writing skills. Ryan has a really hard time holding a pen or pencil and the school seems to make him instead of letting him have use of a computer. He has lots of homework pages to do every night because he can't get them done at school because he writes so slowly. Ryan is very bright and a very lovable child. He has many friends and is enjoyed by everyone.

Cody

Cody was born December 4th, 1993. He was born full term and everything seemed to be OK at first. It was a late delivery and I was really tired when I got back to my room so I did not have him come back in that night. When they brought him to me the next morning, he took my breath away he was so beautiful! When I fed him for the first time, he didn't drink much, and I looked forward to holding him for the rest of the day. But that was cut short because a minute or so after he finished eating he started breathing erratically and I called a nurse immediately. She took him from my arms and out of the room.

From that point on, he was in Special Care Nursery for nine days. They ran all kinds of tests on him, even a drug test without my knowledge. The doctors thought he had water on the lungs, but they really couldn't explain what was causing the erratic and rapid breathing. He was born on a Monday and the doctors were to send us home on Wednesday but when that day came he wanted to keep Cody for one more day, so I talked him into letting me stay till then because Cody had caught on my tailbone and bruised it during birth and I was still hurting pretty bad. But Thursday came and they sent me home without my baby boy. They told me to call back in the morning, which I did. Again the doctor told me just twenty-four more hours. Well this happened over and over again until the following Wednesday. It was very hard on me to keep hearing this every day. If only the doctor could have given me a more honest timeline, instead of getting my hopes up everyday.

Finally, Cody got to come home the following Wednesday and it was so great to have him home. He had a follow up visit scheduled in three weeks. During those three weeks he seemed to not be just right. He wouldn't hold any toys and he always seemed to not be looking at anything. I told the doctor about my thoughts and he checked him thoroughly. He told me that his reflexes were slow, so he decided that Cody needed to have a CT Scan done and he referred me to a neurologist. When the doctor got back the results, he told me that Cody had Dandy Walker variant. I was devastated. All I wanted was a child like my sister had, no problems.

I couldn't understand why this had to happen to me. I did not know anyone that had a child with a disability. I felt so alone. So many questions: why me, how would I handle this, what could have caused this, etc. I cried a lot. As time passed, I felt that this diagnosis was not right. The symptoms did not match up to Dandy Walker.

Most children have hydrocephalus and require a shunt and have cleft lips and underdeveloped arms and legs. This was not Cody. I went to the library and did some research on Dandy Walker and it was just not Cody: he has a very small head, in the 5% range. I could just not believe that we had a correct diagnosis. So when Cody was about 4 months old I decided to go for a second opinion. I chose the second hospital because I was told they dealt with all kinds of diseases, health problems and syndromes and they should be able to help me. So when Cody was five and a half months, my Mother and I traveled out of state to find the answers I was looking for. There they ran test after test, or so it seemed.

They were dumbfounded by Cody's eyes. They didn't know what to think and they wanted me to bring him back in eighteen months. The Pediatric Neurologist told me that he would be fine, all his problem was is that he was missing his vermis and he did not have Dandy Walker variant. It would just take him longer to do things. I was relieved for a little while then as time passed I still had a hard time believing that it was that simple of an answer. There just seemed to be more to it. So while talking to an old friend that I ran into, I found out that she had a child born with a small brain who had had many problems and had since passed. She recommend to me a Pediatric Neurosurgeon, whom I found out later was well known in another city. She believed he could help me. So I made an appointment when Cody was about one year old. He told me, after an examination and looking over his CT scan that he did not have a diagnosis, but Cody definitely had something wrong with him. He went further to say that Cody would never walk or talk and he would be in a wheelchair for the rest of his life. Tears came to my eyes and I left totally devastated. The diagnosis seemed to have gone from bad to better to worse. I was beside myself. How could this happen to me? Why God? I've always felt like I have been a good person and did not deserve such heartache, nor did my little boy. He was so innocent.

A few weeks later I got a telephone call from Cody's neurologist, whom I had thought knew nothing about my searching further for an answer outside of him. He told me that the neurosurgeon called him and they discussed Cody's situation and they came up with Joubert Syndrome. As he spoke to me it was like a calm came over me, my search was over. Everything he described about Joubert Syndrome was Cody: the eye problems, the breathing problems, the developmental delay. After that call I was happy to finally have an answer to what Cody had, yet I was at a loss as to where his future would be going. Right after that call I contacted the National Organization for Rare Disorders and they sent me some information on Joubert Syndrome. On the back there was a name and number for the Joubert Family-In-Touch Network. I remember receiving the information on Halloween and right before I left to take Cody to my friend's house I called that number and spoke to the lady who also had a child with Joubert Syndrome. I didn't feel so alone anymore and everything was better. I talked to her for about one hour and I felt so relieved. My family and friends are very supportive, especially my mother. We are very close and she feels my pain. My husband at the time really had no reaction, he just went with the flow. (Although I felt that he never really accepted that he had a child with a disability. We later divorced right before Cody's second birthday.)

We have been attending Physical, Occupational and Speech Therapy for years. I want to do anything to help my little boy. I still cry a little every now and then when I think about it all, especially when I see a child that is younger than Cody and doing so much more, or when Cody accomplishes a challenge. I used to take the small things for granted but not anymore. Everything that Cody has done from picking up a Cheerio, rolling over, crawling, standing, blowing the candles on his birthday cake to walking have been more pleasurable than I could have ever imagined. We celebrate every little thing and reach for the future with our arms open. I want Cody to experience everything possible.

I used to think that this was a punishment from God for doing something wrong. But now I look at it as a gift. My life has been so enriched by having Cody. He is a great kid and I couldn't have ordered one better. I couldn't imagine life without him. He has brought so much to my life.

The only information I feel that I am missing about Joubert Syndrome is information that I can not get. What does the future hold for my son? Will he be able to grow up and live in a normal atmosphere? Will he be able to adapt to the world? Only time will tell! When someone asks what is wrong with my son. I tell them exactly what it is: he's developmentally delayed due to his brain being underdeveloped and he has definitely come a long way. I would rather someone ask me than to stare and wonder. I feel that I've had more kids ask me what's wrong with his eye than anything (Cody had ptosis of his right eye, before surgery) I would just tell them he was born like that, it doesn't hurt him and he would get it fixed when he got a little older. It's hard to say what the most difficult stage of Cody's development was for me, everything seemed to be a big challenge, from turning over to walking. It's been a rough, yet rewarding, five years. I think it was his walking that was hardest for me. It is such a relief for me now because I do not have to carry him as much, and I was beginning to experience back problems. He feels such a freedom and independence now. We are still working on potty training and that has been a several year battle, but we're still trying. The most difficult stage in Cody's development for him seems to be his fine motor skills. He is so smart. His body wants to do things and he seems to know what he has to do, but he just can't and he gets very mad and throws fits. I want to do everything for him but I realize that if I do he'll never learn for himself. I help as much as I can with what he can't do on his own. I've also realized that I can't put any limitations on him because every time I do, he amazes me and does it. He used to have the same problem with talking to me. I thought about teaching him sign language but I did not think he would be able to, until I went to the biannual Joubert Conference and I met a lady who had a child similar to Cody and she started showing him some sign and he picked up on it so easily, he was only two and a half then. He now uses over one hundred signs to communicate with me and my family. He realizes when other people do not know it and he seems to get across what he wants to say to them by using body language. When he was first learning to use sign, he would only mimic what I did, until about three weeks later. It was late and I wanted to get him to sleep, my niece was staying over and he was hyped up. So I sat down on the couch, picked him up and when I was getting ready to give him the bottle he looked up at me and signed Mommy then Love. He told me that he loved me for the first time. It was so wonderful to finally hear what every mother dreams of hearing. All I could do is hold him and cry.

My main concern about my child's education right now is that he is treated fairly. His teachers are patient with him and can get by without kids teasing him. He's a pretty smart kid so I think he'll learn easily. Right now he is in an Early Childhood Program which caters to special needs children and he loves it. They are very caring and great with him. His teacher seems to think he'll be able to go to a regular kindergarten so they are working on skills he'll need there. The main challenge Cody faces right now is the normal everyday living skills needed. Like pulling down pants to potty, changing his own clothes or shoes, brushing his teeth, getting his own food and drink, etc.

Cody has been through three eye surgeries, two to correct his strabismus (the first did not take) and one on his ptosis, dropping eye lid. That one did not do too well either and he's getting ready to have that fixed again. Putting him through the surgeries has been hard but worth it. He seems to be seeing much better now. He is such a strong child, I only wish I had half of his motivation. I would like to finish with my thought of having a child with a disability. As I said before, I used to think of Cody's disability as a punishment but I've come to realize that it is a gift. God would not have given him to me if I could not have been able to handle it. Please just cherish every moment with your child, even if there is no disability. Life is so short and precious. Every child deserves love and nurturing from their parents.

Sean

Diagnosis Confirmation: 2 days
Present age: 12 yrs
Age of first symptoms: birth

- Sean was originally a foster child that we later adopted—we knew going into this situation there would be significant challenges. He has done better than expected!
- Doctors gave us what little information they had—alll bleak. I felt very isolated since it was so rare. In 12 years I have learned a lot, but there are still mysteries, especially with behaviours. I hope the gene will be discovered.
- I am pretty gregarious and pro-active—I usually initiate the conversation, so telling them about Sean flows naturally. I describe Joubert Syndrome, the adventure of raising Sean, and the Network/Foundation.
- Around 1–2yrs, teething resulted in serious self injurious behaviour (biting lip and hand) Also recently (12 yrs) increased head banging.
- We have an excellent school system and the staff peo-

ple (teachers, aides, PT OT + S/L) are like family—we are blessed! We are all "in the dark" about reading potential as Sean is inconsistent in his responses.

- Sean lives at home and attends Public School. One of the biggest challenges is the self-abusive behaviour and obstinacy when it comes to learning activities. We are all creative, but he has always shown great "task avoidance" ability. We are anxious to tap into the intelligence we know is there.

Fanny

- Her head was too small at birth (31cm). At 3 months, I thought she was kind of slow; at 5 months, she still did not touch any object; at 6 months, I was desperate that someone tell me what was wrong with her general lack of interest and motivation.
- After 3½ years, we still do not accept the situation. Our life was so beautifully planned and now that dream has been crushed. One thing has not changed though: our incredible love for our daughter.
- I was just scared that she might die and felt relieved that she was just handicapped, until I came to realize the impact of that fact and the hard work it involved and would involve for the rest of our lives.
- We saw a neurologist when she was 3 years old who invoked the possibility of Joubert Syndrome.
- Whatever the syndrome, it won't change the situation.

I am just relieved to know that she will not necessarily die on me, that she might be able to walk, etc. In fact, only time will tell how she will progress.

- I went to the symposium in Montreal and got a lot of information there. It was extremely informative and answered many of my questions.
- That she is handicapped and is probably affected by Joubert Syndrome, which affects her eyes, her breathing, her tone and her general development.
- To take an interest in toys, to touch them and to be able to move around.
- She is not very old, but I think it will be to communicate her needs.
- I will be satisfied if they teach her to be the most autonomous possible. I also hope they will be able to teach her how to effectively communicate her needs.
- For the moment, I am teaching her myself with the help of the therapists and I am presently looking for the best school for her.
- To realize she is not the only one on this planet who has needs. To let other people than Mom and Dad feed her, teach her things. To get out of the house, be with other people at different places, interact with other kids and adults.

Antoine

Country: France
Diagnosis confirmed: 10 months
Age of first symptoms: 3 months
Present age: 2 years

- Antoine could not hold his head properly when he was three months old. Moreover, he could not follow the light and seemed not to be able to see very well.

- We were very anxious because it took seven months to know that he was suffering from Joubert Syndrome. We then tried to learn about the disease and what it would mean for Antoine's future. As he was our first and only child, we did not know if he was late in his development compared to unaffected children.

  The rest of the family was also very anxious and understood rather quickly that the disease was very serious.

- The doctors in here were the ones who first diagnosed the syndrome when Antoine was ten months old. Without any explanation whatsoever, we asked for further information in Paris. We really understood what the Joubert syndrome was about once we received some information from the Parents-in-Touch Network from the States. Then, we met Professor Boltshauser in Zurich.

- At that time, we had great difficulty accepting the syndrome and we hoped that Antoine would not suffer too much. Now, we know that Antoine is not severely affected by the syndrome, and we do our best to make him happy and to help him make some good progress in order to be autonomous.

- We have collected much information concerning JS itself, which is rather technical for us, but we lack information concerning the way children cope with the disease, how we should handle it and how to help them properly. The most important question for us is to know how Antoine will be in ten to twenty years time.
- Although it is always very painful for us, we clearly explain what's wrong with our child and why he is different. In the same time, we must admit that it is difficult at first sight to see that Antoine is suffering from any disease, that's why people don't ask many questions.
- What's most important for us is to know whether Antoine will be able to walk and talk as he has some difficulty now.
- Antoine seems to feel frustrated as he would like to walk and to make him understand and he cannot do it.
- We would like to know if Antoine will be able to attend school normally or if he will have to go to a special school. Moreover, we don't know how he will manage to cope with school, learnings and activities. But our main concern is are there any good and adapted schools for our child in our hometown or in any other place?
- Antoine is too young to go to school. He goes to a kindergarten and will carry on until he is three years old. After that, he might be able to go to a nursery

school. In the meantime, we spend a lot of time stimulating him by as many activities as possible. Antoine loves doing things like drawing, cooking, doing like us, reading, playing with his legos, etc.

- Will he talk? Will he walk? Will he keep progressing and most important, will he always be as happy as he seems to be now?

  We would also like to know how those children evolve, how they will react when they are grown-ups.

- Antoine is mostly at home. He goes to a kindergarten three to four times a week. He goes to a physiotherapist twice a week, once to an orthoptist (for his eyes) and once to a speech therapist. I have stopped working to be with him as much as possible and to stimulate him by doing all sorts of activities.

- Antoine is willing to communicate and he is doing his best to be understood by showing us things, by pronouncing sounds that are more and more understandable.

  He is not able to walk although he is able to make a few steps, but he uses a big truck to move in the flat and he is able to go wherever he wants.

Rossana

Because of language barriers, this family in Italy submits a point form discussion of their daughter's development instead of a story. It amazes me how many similarities there are between these individuals all over the world.

91/08/20 Birth date.

92/09 She follows objects with both eyes; seldom she control the head(from prone position). She catches objects to her mouth.

93/01 She controls the head, catches objects (better with left hand).

93/06 She sits by herself for short time (seconds) with frontal hands support. She stays on all fours for several seconds. She catches objects in the middle.

94/02 She sits by herself also with back balance.
She makes exercises on her weight with the help of physiotherapist.

94/09 She starts to tell sounds to communicate. She sends kisses. She starts to lean on her hands.She sits by her sides too. She keep the kneeling positions with frontal support.

95/01 She rolls with help from back(supine) to sitting position. She has side support reactions(better on right side). She keeps the side sitting position. From this position she proceeds to kneeling position if she has a front support. She uses better the hands to take and to throw away objects. But she has shakes and dissymetry.

She uses static table. To sustain the weight, she uses orthopedic shoes.

95/11 Good balance in sitting position. She rolls. She tries to skid on feet position from the sofa. She starts to stay for 30 seconds on kneeling position.

96/04 She has improved the balance on kneeling position. She proceeds from side sitting position to kneeling position. She uses spontaneously the hands to pass objects from one hand to another. First expressive gestures (she says hello with the hand).

96/05 Exercises to stand erect and to walk.

She moves forward without bending her knees but only with the rush of legs.

96/08 She starts to use bicycle, she does not pedal but she is pushed by someone.

96/10 Start of horse riding therapy (once a week for half an hour).

96/11 Start of speech therapy (once a week for 45 minutes).

Start of occupational therapy (once a week for 1 hour).

96/12 Start of swimming therapy (once a week for 45 minutes).

97/01 Start of school (kindergarten) with children of 4/5 years old.

She starts to walk by herself with one person behind, keeping her shoulders.

97/03 She starts to have long speeches (ba-ba-ba -ma ma-ma).

97/05 She knows objects, pictures. She has long distance memory. She knows colors.

97/07 She uses “logical blocks”, she knows colors and shapes. She can select a particular shape, thick or thin, with a particular color.

97/08 Using the bycicle she try to pedals by herself for about 100 m.

She use bicycle for more than an hour.

97/09 School again with children 4/5 years old. She start to drink using the glass (held by another).

97/10 She answers (with usual ba-ba-ba...) to complex questions (images-ideas association, i.e. ex.).

97/11 She says yes and no with the head.

97/12 She stands by herself when if she does not notice it.

She walks assisted, when interested.

PRESENT SITUATION 6/98 age: 6 years 10 months

SPEECH

- only ba-ba , ma-ma, pa, pe
- beginning of words with pi , no, ta
- we have to propose her different alternatives (list of words/action) . She says yes or no with the head
- she gives complex answers (not understandable, ba-ba-me-me-ma-ma repeated) to our questions
- often she keeps her fingers into the mouth

- she keeps in a good way the mouth shut
- no/few blows
- she gives kisses
- she crunch well
- no sucking with straws

PHYSICAL

- she uses both hands also with little object
- she passes objects from an hand to another
- she leafs through the book pages
- she walks assisted with rigid legs for 120 meters each time (when she wants)
- she goes on stairs (assisted)
- she stands by herself (for almost three minutes)

BEHAVIOUR

- she accepts other unknown people (at distance). When near she puts hands around her head.
- she weeps when there are unexpected people or strong emotions.
- she accept children at short distance.
- she makes bye with hands to all (without request).
- very hard problems to dress/undress her. She tries not to make her dress/undress with cries and moving her body.
- when she wants something she tries with all her forces (cries, refusal of alternative).
- she is stubborn.
- she is habitual, she uses to do the same things with the same persons.
- she does activities (walking, etc.) when attracted by food.

- she prefers to stay sit or stand watching children to play than to play by herself.
- she is very curious. She wants to control everything happens in a room or around her (when outside).
- She uses diapers.
- She does not eat or drink by herself, but she takes little piece of food and feed herself. When she is thirsty, she takes the glass trying to drink.

Dessert

Erin, again

Erin

We went camping the summer of Erin's sixth birthday at Rondeau Park. What a wonderful time we had! The second day there, Erin lost her first two baby teeth: one in a piece of chocolate cake at lunch and the other on a Dorito by the campfire. The tooth fairy found us, of course, and although Erin had absolutely insisted that the tooth fairy brought ten dollars, she was satisfied with the three loonies she found in her pillowcase the next morning.

The hardest part of the week was Erin having her first "boy friend". Matthew was camping with his family next door and at nine years of age, still enjoyed the slower and quieter things in life. Perhaps because he was third of four children he reminded me of Kevin: he enjoyed "belly botany", reading and spoke excitedly of Shel Silverstein's *Where the Sidewalk Ends.* He and Erin played with toys on a blanket, read books, and talked. Erin told us Matthew was cool. He told his mom Erin was his new best friend.

It was a landmark event for me (and I'm sure for Erin, too!) I was shown that there are definitely people her age that would understand her and want to be a part of her life. I'm sure I'll always worry about her, but that's my job. I'm her mom. I wonder if I'm doing the right thing, making the right decisions, doing....enough. OH, and of course I still have to decide what make for supper.

Maybe we'll have stew tonight.

Appendices

Appendix A: Joubert Syndrome Foundation FAQ

All information is gathered from the website: www.joubertfoundation.com and is reprinted with permission.

What is Joubert Syndrome?

Joubert Syndrome is a very rare genetic disorder in which there are congenital problems which fit into a recognizable pattern of features.

What are the characteristics of Joubert Syndrome?

The most typical features of Joubert Syndrome include:

- Absence or underdevelopment of part of the brain called the cerebellum vermis which controls balance and coordination.
- A malformed brain stem, which may cause an abnormal breathing pattern called episodic hypernea, in which babies pant, and may be followed by apnea (cessation of breathing).
- Abnormal eye and tongue movements.
- Decreased muscle tone. It can be marked in the neonatal period and in infancy.
- Seizures (less typical).

How is Joubert Syndrome inherited?

Joubert Syndrome is inherited in an autosomal recessive manner. Both parents are carriers of the gene. Genetic testing is not currently available to detect this condition. Parents who have a child with Joubert Syndrome have a 1 in 4 chance of having another affected child in another pregnancy. Prenatal testing with a level 3 ultrasound may be possible.

What is the prognosis for Joubert Syndrome?

While global and developmental delay is frequent, health and growth are usually not severely affected. Commonly there is a degree of mild or moderate retardation. Severe mental retardation is uncommon. There are a few cases of affected individuals with normal intelligence or learning abilities.

What is the treatment for Joubert Syndrome?

Infant stimulation, physical therapy, occupational therapy, and speech therapy are valuable. Somewhat less traditional therapies such as auditory training, sensory integration, horseback therapy and water therapy have also been found to be very beneficial. Infants with abnormal breathing should have apnea monitoring.

Common Abnormalities:

Muscle tone: Hypotonia present in all patients. It can be marked in the neonatal period and in infancy.

Balance: Approximately 75% of children learn to sit and 50% learn to walk. Sitting occurs at approximately 18 months and walking occurs at 4 years. Assistance is required to complete kneeling to stand transition.

Extreme calcaneal eversion is noted when standing. Gait is unstable and tandem walking is poor.

Development: Developmental delay is present across a variety of domains including adaptive behaviors, motor, language, and general development. Children are pleasant, friendly, easy to guide, and socially well integrated. Developmental delay is often severe.

Neuroradiology: A MRI scan shows molar tooth sign in axial plane; deeper than normal posterior interpeduncular fossa, prominent or thickened superior cerebellar penduncles, and vermis hypoplasia or dysplasia. MRI in coronal and axial planes show clefting of the vermis. MRI in sagittal plane shows abnormally shaped and rostrally displaced fourth ventricle.

Pathology: Vermis hypoplasia or displasia, elongation of the caudal midbrain tegmentum, and marked dysplasia of the caudal medulla.

Associated Abnormalities:

Face: High rounded eyebrows, broad nasal bridge and mild epicanthus, antiverted nostrils, triangular shaped open mouth with irregular tongue protrusion, low set coarse ears.

Breathing: Episodic hyperpnea and/or apnea in 50–75% of patients. Breathing abnormalities most pronounced in the neonatal period and in infancy.

Eyes: Retinal dysplasia, colobomas, nystagmus, strabismus, and ptosis. Retinal blindness is rarely present.

Ocular-motor: Apraxia and vestibulo-ocular cancellation/pursuit defects.

Renal: Microcystic renal disease may be progressive.

Limbs: Polydactyly may be present.

Uncommon: Macrocephaly, Microcephaly, esophageal reflux, soft tissue tongue tumors, epilepsy, congenital heart defects, duodenal atresia, choanal atresia, ocular fibrosis, liver anomalies, pectus excavatum, Hirschsprung's disease, vocal cord paralysis and occipital meningocele.

Mail the foundation at:

12348 Summer Meadow Rd.
Rock, MI 49880
attn: Mary Van Damme
Telephone: 906-359-4707

or contact

Cheryl Duquette
Joubert Syndrome Foundation President
410-997-8084

Appendix B: Map of the Human Brain

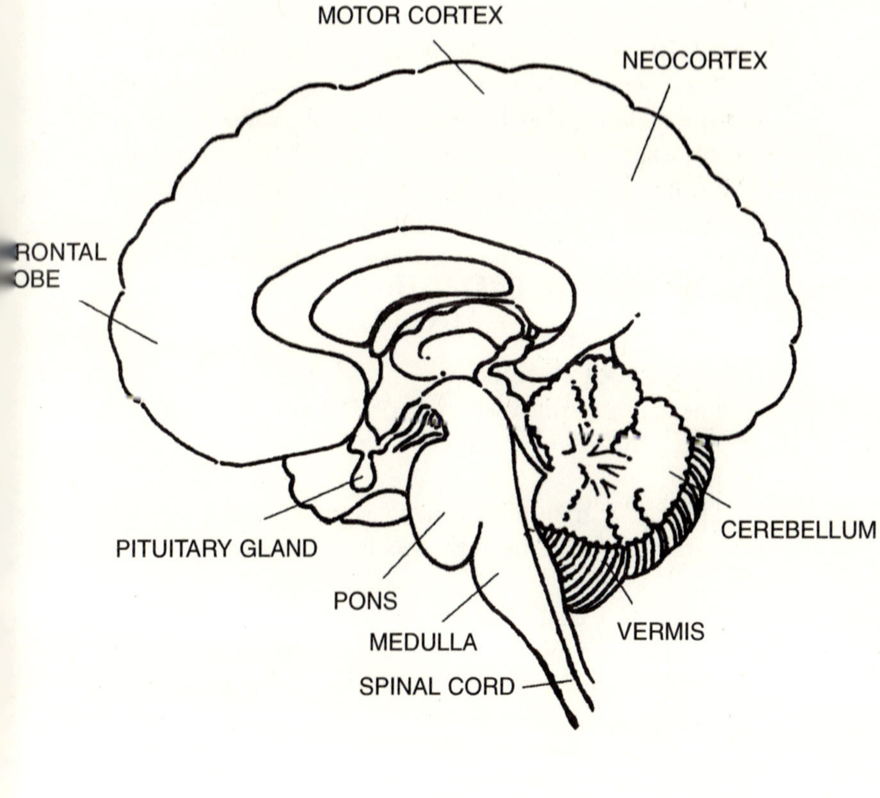

This sketch of the brain by Judith Reisman has been a staple in many of Bonnie Hanschu's courses. It appears here with permission from Bonnie.

Appendix C: Sensory Processing Therapy Report for Erin

When I began using sensory processing therapy with Erin, I tried to be as "detached" as possible in order to evaluate whether this was really "working" or whether I was just seeing what I wanted. The following is a detailed report that I kept during that time. It now serves as a case study to demonstrate the effectiveness of this type of therapy for Erin.

READY APPROACH: ASSESSMENT 1 —AUG 18/98

Discussion of Results

There is an indication in 3 of 4 areas (all but proprioception) the Erin is exhibiting signs of sensory defensiveness.

There is a strong pattern of signs of registration and integration problems in the vestibular and proprioceptive areas.

There is a question of whether Erin is truly having modulation problems. Although she definitely has problems with many types of transitions, all other indicators are questionable at this time.

Treatment Plan

The Wilbarger Protocol will be administered beginning August 19, 1998.

A sensory diet rich in vestibular and proprioceptive input will also begin at that time. Tactile opportunities will continue to be incorporated as done prior to this inventory with emphasis on better timing and diversity to support the Wilbarger Protocol.

Extra "doses" of proprioception are to be administered before and during key transition periods, specifically, between environments (in and out of house, car, etc.) and before eating.

Vestibular and proprioceptive input should be administered in a slow, strong and repetitive way until Erin is able to handle more complex input.

Baseline behaviours—Aug '98

- can't find the "right words"
- hits out (at others, at air)
- throws toys
- refuses to walk on feet
- paints mouth with tongue
- afternoon "meltdown"
- stuffs mouth with food

Follow-up Notes

Aug 19 Day 1

- began brushing protocol
- "paint and find" feet and hands every 1½ hours
- cooperated completely by 3rd brushing (held her down for first two)
- blood work done—high trauma
- no change in baseline behaviours
- no other changes observed

Aug 20 Day 2

- seems more upset and angry all day, resistant to normal routine

- increase in baseline
- "I Love You" song seemed more musical today, not all one tone
- no bowel movement

Aug 21 Day 3

- same as Day 2, still no bowel movement

Aug 22 Day 4

- bowel movement
- began swinging program—especially responsive to bounce and circle
- missed 3:30 brush due to trauma—cut hand: cut didn't bother her but screamed for 20 minutes as we tried to clean it, ended up with no bandage until bedtime
- increased mid-line control: held yogurt cup with one hand while spoon feeding with other, used two hands to get melon cube on fork

Aug 23 Day 5

- quite upset when taking Band-Aid off
- drawing seems disorganized
- enjoyed swing but became agitated when rotated
- responded well to wrap and cuddle with soothing music

Aug 24 Day 6

- resistant to brushing/compression—says compressions hurt
- agitated during swing rotation but insists that you continue, recommend no rotational swinging for the next while

- slight decrease in baseline
- no afternoon meltdown in last 3–4 days

Aug 25 Day 7

- brushing and swinging went well
- added ankle weight when walking
- informing us when she has wet/soiled her diaper

Aug 26 Day 8

- mom sick—brushing only

Aug 27 Day 9

- excellent results in hitting out and throwing
- improvement in general language: seems quicker and more appropriate in responses i.e. Kev: (in kitchen to Erin at TV) "Erin, come here!" Erin: "Coming!" (moves to door) "What?" —very "normal" and not something she's done before
- walked in to CRC for appt with Toni—walker and ankle weights—stride was quick at times, left foot turned in when bringing forward

Aug 28 Day 10

- still not drawing/writing, just scribbles

Aug 29 Day 11

- Excellent day! Behaviour generally more easily regulated (2 late night in a row with early mornings but no real meltdowns—one 15 minute period of irritation and hitting out but calmed down and rest of day was good)
- posture noticeably better in sitting
- played board game and followed the play herself

almost to the end of game
- drew a picture—no scribbles

Aug 30 Day 12
- notice that she will come to another room to tell me something about what she is doing, then return to the task after the report is over

Aug 31 Day 13
- went shopping at the mall for 2nd day in a row and no meltdown on the way home in car!

Sept 1 Day 14
- beginning to attempt some consonant sounds in her speech
- some agitation and "wrong word choice" in morning but rest of day was good
- imaginative play has grown—used to simply dress and undress dolls, noticed in last few days that Erin has them talking to each other, or playing with a toy dog or taking care of a baby doll
- informed us that she was wet and wanted to be changed
- chose a bedtime book in hardly any time with no meltdown

Two Week Summary

As in any new therapy, there was hope that changes would be more obviously dramatic but none of her baseline behaviours were extremely severe either. The changes we have seen are exciting and gratifying and it wasn't until they changed that we realized how significant they were. She is generally more content, responsive, initiates conversation, gives detail in her reports, recovers from agitations more easily and is more aware of her self and environment.

Sept 2 Day 15

- some agitation in the morning but was able to manage it
- asked for a "cuddle wrap" in afternoon—was getting agitated just before
- noted that her sleep seems less restless, not moving around bed as much, in the last few nights

Sept 3 Day 16

- Kevin reported good day
- as we were reading a book, a video tape ended its rewind cycle, Erin immediately went over, ejected the tape and put it into its case!
- some problems settling to sleep (but Sarah was also awake!)

Three Week Summary

This past week has been good. Erin seems to be short tempered but recovers well, sometimes without any help. We are still brushing every 1½ hours, swinging 1–2x a day and adding leg weights, bed-bouncing, cuddle-wraps, wrestling and anything else we can think of as often as possible. She seemed more sound-sensitive on the 5th and 6th but has not seemed bothered since. The latest "milestone" occurred on Sept 9 (today) when Erin chewed a piece of gum for over an hour. Traditionally, it was swallowed within 3 minutes. Baseline behaviours are infrequent and less severe than before treatment began. We are cutting down the brushing/compression regimen to 3x a day over the next 4 days in preparation for school. We will continue as much of the sensory diet as possible with the 3 brushings remaining as part of that diet.

Two Month Summary

Erin continues to do extremely well. Some notable firsts include:

- reporting pain during her latest ear infection;
- wiping her ear when it was draining from the infection;
- waking in the night to tell us she was cold—and then going back to sleep;
- increase in duration while walking;
- more easily calmed after being upset or overwhelmed;
- increase in motivation to have speech understood and working harder at consonant sounds;

There have been concerns that she has "lost ground" in the past month especially in the area of maintaining equilibrium. We attribute that to not having as much intervention as we would have liked in the first three weeks of school and her general health. We now have a better schedule which includes 4 brushings, 2–3 swings, 2 sessions with ankle weights, weighted vest at mid-day and incidental (not scheduled) wrestling, cuddle wraps, push-ups, etc. as needed.

The SII will be re-administered in one month and the sensory diet will be adjusted as necessary.

Four Month Summary

These past two months have been difficult. We have

been without an in-home worker since October and there have been problems with consistency at the school. There has been no continuity of program and there has been resulting regression. We are seeing a reappearance of baseline behaviours with a new one—perseveration (task and speech). I have contacted Laura Barker and she will be assessing Erin using my information and her own and will consult with us re: Erin's program. The SII will be re-administered in preparation for this meeting.

READY APPROACH: ASSESSMENT 2 —DEC 29/98

Discussion of Results

There is an indication in 3 of 4 areas (all but proprioception) the Erin is exhibiting signs of sensory defensiveness. These indicators are not as strong as the first inventory, nor do we see the behaviours as often as before. Nonetheless, they are still present.

There continues to be a strong pattern of signs of registration and integration problems in the vestibular and proprioceptive areas. Again, the indicators are not as strong/often as before.

The question of whether Erin is truly having modulation problems is still present although I consider it less likely. Although she definitely has problems with some types of transitions, all other indicators are questionable at this time.

Overall Observations

When completing the SII this time, it was noted that the frequency and severity of "yes" responses was milder than during the first inventory. It was still somewhat discouraging to see little surface change within the inventory results.

This past week has given us more observation time. Several things have been noted:

- as well as continuing to chew gum, she will now indicate when it is stuck on a tooth and can locate it with fingers to throw it out
- seems to need more "calming wraps" than pre-December (or perhaps, we use the technique more readily)
- has resumed "normal" night habits—even breathing, less restless—since the December disruption
- we have gotten better at administering extra doses of proprioception and deep pressure before car/meal transitions. Although it was in the original treatment plan, we did not find it necessary to be diligent about it until the "December disruption"
- has a tendency to perseverate after using the v-swing (HAS to watch an episode of Arthur)

Treatment Plan

The plan will be updated following the Jan 29 consultation with Laura Barker.

Plan was continued with only a few minor changes:

- Laura demonstrated a more efficient and faster way to utilize the swing
- demonstrated and encouraged the use of the oral element of the Wibarger Protocol

Laura was extremely helpful and supportive during her visit. It made us feel like we really were making a difference and that we were on the right track. It is hard to remember that when you are in the middle of the routine.

READY APPROACH: ASSESSMENT 3 —August 5, 1999

Discussion of Results

Erin's vestibular and proprioception continue to need attention especially in the areas of registration and integration. There has been definite progress made however. She no longer lays her head on the table to colour or watch TV. Her posture has improved in all areas and she joins in to physical activities with little or no prompting. She is more aware of and able to maneuver herself into balanced positions on furniture and maintains a better grasp on most objects.

Her greatest gain is in the area of emotional outbursts. Whereas last year they were frequent, unpredictable and prolonged (sometimes 1-4 hours) her responses now seem to have a definite trigger and rarely last more than 15-20 minutes, usually just 5 minutes.

There is now a much clearer picture of Erin. The areas of need are more obviously consistent with a person who has neuromotor problems. Her global defensiveness is now reduced to a sensitivity to sound (which has improved as of Sept 3,199!), a sensitivity to some direct light and touching cold temperatures—and having her toenails cut!

Erin stopped bringing her wheelchair to school in late March. She manages her day with her walker quite well. She works very hard at producing clear speech. She still separates many sounds within a word and her syntax is...unique (close to ASL grammar). Personal pronouns are beginning to emerge and breath control is increasing.

Baseline Behavioral Report—Sept '99

- can't find the "right words" —rarely seen
- hits out (at others, at air)—seen only during overload
- throws toys—rarely seen
- refuses to walk on feet—resolved
- paints mouth with tongue—rarely seen (usually during a cold)
- afternoon "meltdown"—seen but controlled
- stuffs mouth with food—usually

The typeface chosen for this book is
ITC Galliard, which was adapted from a
1978 design by Matthew Carter for Mergenthaler.
The typeface was modeled on the work of
the 16th century letter cutter, Robert Granjon.

The book was designed by David Langs.

The book was printed and bound by AGMV Marquis in
Montreal, Quebec, Canada.

AGMV Marquis
MEMBER OF THE SCABRINI GROUP
Quebec, Canada
2001